Ethics: The Heart of Health Care

David Seedhouse
Departments of Community Health and General Practice
The University of Liverpool
Liverpool, UK

JOHN WILEY & SONS
Chichester · New York · Brisbane · Toronto · Singapore

Copyright © 1988 by John Wiley & Sons Ltd.

Reprinted October 1989
Reprinted March 1991

Distributed in the United States of America, Canada and Japan by Alan R. Liss Inc.,
41 East 11th Street, New York, NY 10003, USA.

Library of Congress Cataloging-in-Publication Data:

Seedhouse, David
  Ethics: the heart of health care
  (A Wiley medical publication)
  Bibiliography: p.
  Includes index.
  1. Medical ethics.   I. Title.   II. Series.
R724.S43 1988   174'.2   87-37253
ISBN 0 471 91874 1 (pbk.)

British Library Cataloguing in Publication Data:

Seedhouse, David
  Ethics: the heart of health care
  1. Health services. Ethical aspects
  I. Title
  174'.2

  ISBN 0 471 91874 1

Printed in Great Britain at the Alden Press, Oxford

Ethics: The Heart of
Health Care

For Simon and Mary Elstow

'Will somebody pass me the bloody salt ... please?'—Dennis, from his armchair, 1988.

A person's optimum state of heath is equivalent to the state of the set of conditions which fulfil or enable a person to work to fulfil his or her realistic chosen and biological potentials.—Seedhouse 1986.

In his novel *Nineteen Eighty Four*, George Orwell describes four Ministries through which 'The Party' holds power: a Ministry of Peace concerned with war, a Ministry of Love for law and order, a Ministry of Plenty to deal with scarcities, and a Ministry of Truth where a vast system of brain washing is carried out. He did not need to describe a Ministry of Health which deals with disease because we already have one.—Wilson 1976.

Contents

Acknowledgements

During the period in which this book was created my life took on a life of its own. This was a strange and crazy life which refused to tell me what it intended to do next, or why. Fortunately this other life never found out about the book. I deeply thank Alan Cribb and Annmarie Carlen for helping me keep the secret.

Both these friends were of immense practical help, as were Harry Lesser and Mary Brown. The Departments of Community Health and General Practice at Liverpool University kindly allowed me the necessary time to write the book, and the Health Education Authority allowed me the necessary money to pay my bills.

There were various influences on my other life which must also be acknowledged. My other life would like to thank Ulrig and Martha from Metz for introducing it to a novel sport, Gabby from Florence for introducing it to the Italian version of Teutonic efficiency, and Luxembourg for not being any bigger. Thanks are also due to Chrissie Adams (Zandra Rhodes under a cobalt sky with Standards), my lawyer, Chorlton Water Park, the Nitromors Co., and an ever-circling squabble of dingoes for continuing to circle. Further gratitude is due to 16 December 1986, 20 February, 28 April, and 26 September 1987, and to Frank and the boys for not designing the cover to this book. There will always be a special place in the heart of my other life for Duffy Seedhouse. Although this boy is now ten years old he has never once uttered a word of complaint or protest.

Preface

This book extends a theory about the nature of health into the heart of practice. It is genuinely philosophy applied. And it is long overdue.

In the majority of areas of human activity there exist theories, sometimes a range of competing theories, about the meaning of a particular activity, about its limits, about the sorts of methods and techniques that are most suited to it, about its implications for other areas of activity, and about the moral issues that are raised by it. Such theories are usually known as philosophies. So not only are there specific human activities known as medicine and social science, for instance, but there are also branches of inquiry which try to analyse and understand the rationale of the practices.

Thus there is a philosophy of medicine and a philosophy of social science which aim at uncovering the *raison d'être* of each discipline. Since the philosophies are concerned with the underlying reasons for the practical activities so they inevitably have an influence on the future development of them. Work within the philosophy of medicine may ask, for instance, whether treatments in medicine should be given *at any cost*, or whether there are occasions on which it is better not to treat patients. The philosophy of social science asks questions about what forms of inquiry are truly to count as social science, and about how much faith can be placed in the reliability of any results generated from inquiry in social science. The answers offered in response to such theoretical questions can have immense practical impact on the parent activities.

It is, at first sight, puzzling that there is no discipline concerned with the philosophy of health. Given that health work periodically affects every member of society (at least in the Western world) from a time before birth until death it is surprising that so little attention has been given to its philosophy. A partial explanation for this phenomenon is that 'health work' is a term with such a wide variety of meanings and applications—from open-heart surgery to political action over environmental hazards—that it is extremely difficult to identify it as a single coherent body of activity. Also, many of the constituent parts of health work—such as medicine and social science—already have their own philosophies.

However, it has been shown (Seedhouse 1986) that health work can be delineated—albeit within a broad boundary—and that this process of delineation and clarification can have implications for practice. For instance, some forms of practice—say, drug trials carried out on patients without their knowledge—can be seen to be work for health in only a very limited sense, if at all. And other practices not normally considered to be work for health—say, talking to a person to help him picture his social circumstances in a more realistic way—can now be seen to be work for health in a very strong sense. Clarification can change the priorities of practice.

Ethics: The Heart of Health Care further pioneers the exploration of the philosophy of health. By charting the extent to which moral issues permeate work for health, by demonstrating tangibly and graphically that *work for health is truly a moral endeavour*, a solid and useful theoretical basis for health workers of all kinds is created. From this platform health workers can grasp more firmly the theoretical significance of their everyday activities. Having gained a stronger grasp on theory health workers are placed in a far better position to appreciate the extent to which they have a huge personal responsibility for the health care they give. Such responsibility is frequently demanding and trying, but if it is handled with confidence it can also be exciting and fulfilling.

The Argument of the Book—Philosophy Applied

It is time that philosophy is again recognized for what it is. Philosophy is an essential part of the way in which we understand our world. It is a process of inquiry that can have real practical effect. The best philosophers are not happy merely to 'watch the wheels turn'. They know that what they do can help produce better wheels, or even rearrange those wheels so that a different machine is created. Philosophy can rejuvenate practice.

This book makes the following points and connections. It forms a powerful guide for those in health care who wish to work with a high degree of morality, and who would also like to improve the structure and organization of health care.

- The world of health care is undergoing a period of intellectual crisis, quite separate from the current political and economic debates on the funding and cost-effectiveness of the NHS. There are a number of forces that are challenging existing assumptions and patterns of practice. These forces include rising interest in holistic medicine; increasing pressure by lay people to have access to medical secrets, including their own medical records; pressure to include the study of medical ethics in undergraduate curricula; and the arguments of some social scientists and health promoters that work for health must begin in society rather than focus on individuals.

- The tension between old and new ideas can be illustrated by an idea borrowed from the philosophy of science—the notion of 'paradigm shift'. It is best to think of this notion only as an analogy rather than a reality. The old paradigm—the old set of cherished beliefs and principles—is being called into question by the new forces. Hence a period of crisis exists in which conflicting ideas and principles do metaphorical battle.

  The process of change from one paradigm to another is not definite and predictable. The future must, to an extent, be shaped actively by people. The question is: *How is it possible to ensure that the new era of health care that emerges from the period of crisis has the best possible form and content*?

- The route to an answer is opened up by offering health workers a more comprehensive understanding of the nature of ethics. Ethics is the key to the new era of health care. Health workers must know that *work for health is a moral endeavour*.

- But work for health is not a moral endeavour in the sense of a crusade. It is not a moral endeavour in an evangelical sense. The task is not to identify what is good and bad, right and wrong, as a dogmatist might. Ethics is not a discipline in which pure blacks and whites can be uncovered and then applied for ever without further question. Ethics is always a question of degree, a question of deliberating about which interventions in other people's lives will produce the highest possible degree of morality.

• But how can the degree of morality of an intervention be assessed in any objective sense? Both ethics and health work are beset by the problem that people in complex societies have different values and beliefs. What one person believes to be a good intervention in the life of another, an intervention exhibiting a high degree of morality, another person might regard as a poor intervention. Even advice about diet and exercise is never based wholly on fact. At some stage a value judgement of some kind will be made.

The extent of the influence of value judgement can be seen from the ten case studies presented in Chapter Four. There are no clear-cut solutions to any of the situations presented, and whatever solution is proposed must involve some reference to values.

Since people's values frequently conflict, how, if at all, can a firm theoretical basis for consistent moral intervention be given to which all health workers can assent?

• There is a range of answers which fail.

(1) One might search for the 'objectively good'. In other words one might pursue some ultimate value or ordering of values which is truly moral. But there can be no means of uncovering the 'truly moral' since in ethics much depends upon personal opinion and subjective judgement. It is not possible to discover the 'objectively good' as one might discover Mount Everest, or a solution to a problem in applied mathematics.

(2) Alternatively, one might search for a set of rules, or a code of practice, to provide a firm uncontroversial basis. However, experience shows that whatever rule, or set of rules, is selected there are always exceptions. There will always be courses of action which offend the rules but lead to the creation of a higher degree of morality than if the rules had been obeyed.

(3) One might appeal to law, but a similar problem to that of the appeal to rules arises.

(4) Or one might instead settle for a relativist position, where it is accepted that there is no objective standard of morality, where what is to be done depends upon judgements made at the time under the existing circumstances. The trouble with this option is that morality can become a meaningless term. Given sufficient advocacy any form of intervention might become permissible for a time. Current law might prohibit some actions, but the higher court of appeal—the court of morality—will be left powerless.

• Where is the foundation for consistent moral intervention to be found? An appeal has to be made to the facts about human nature and potential. Although it is very hard to determine what a truly good human potential or action is, it is less difficult to establish which actions are truly bad. It can be shown that certain ways of limiting human beings—ways of *dwarfing* people mentally, physically, and spiritually—are plainly immoral. Consequently, moves to prevent *dwarfing*, examples of attempts to liberate the enhancing potentials that people possess, form a basis for the most moral health work.

- How can this assertion be given support? Attention has to be paid to the definition of 'personhood'. What is a person, and what forms of human potential, out of all the possibilities, are the most important and significant? The view is advanced that the mental life of a person, which forms an essential part of the definition of 'personhood', is at least as important a target for health work as a person's physical life.

- It is important that health workers are in a position to apply the results of this analysis. So, with relevant and accessible examples, traditional theories of moral philosophy are explained. Too often in the past these theories have been left to languish in a scholarly vacuum.

- However, even with this theoretical background and firm base, there remains much uncertainty and room for conflicts of values within the ethics of health. But this is simply the nature of ethics. *The* right course of action cannot be prescribed as if it were a pill for a specific ill. There will always be legitimate alternative courses of action that might be chosen.

- Because of this constant need for deliberation and balancing of principles, a tool—the *Ethical Grid*—is offered to health workers both as an illustration of the nature of moral reasoning and as an aid to choosing actions to produce the highest degree of morality. Through the use of this tool health workers have the means to justify their choices, to explain how these choices might be shown to be the most strongly opposed to *dwarfing*.

  The Ethical Grid is not a calculating machine. It is merely a euphemism for 'ethical reflection'. It can produce different solutions to the same situation dependent upon who is using it (that is to say, dependent upon who is deliberating). But it does enable health workers to be clear about what is immoral by indicating the range of interventions which lie beyond the limits of the grid. And by giving a clear core rationale the grid allows health workers a basis on which to decide for themselves between alternative possible interventions.

- Finally, recalling the ideas of crisis, paradigm change, and ethics as a key, some implications for the future of health care are considered. Principles such as 'respect for autonomy' and 'respect people as equals' have become likely new priorities for health work. If these principles, and others contained within the core of the grid, are accepted by those with the power to alter the shape of health care, then it will take on a different form. One possible new structure amongst many alternatives is sketched out to show how philosophical investigation—the process of clarification coupled with proposals generated out of logical analysis—can carry true practical weight.

Here, at last, are the beginnings of a philosophy of health.

Part I

'Work for health is a moral endeavour'

Chapter One
Growing Pains

In the Midst of Crisis

The world of health is in crisis. This particular crisis is not financial. The turmoil which surrounds the health professions has swelled because of conceptual confusion. The meaning of the word 'health' has again come under close scrutiny, and it has become clear that the notions of *health* and *human value* are inseparable. Since the idea of health is always associated with the idea of value, and since people frequently have different values, it is possible to advocate a wide variety of aims for health work and a health service, each of which could be justified in various ways. This raises pressing questions: How can a decision be made about which aims should be foremost? How can health work be justified in ethical terms? How can health work be organized and performed so as to produce the greatest benefits for all? What prices should be paid in order to ensure the fruition of the richest sense of health? It is only by addressing these major questions comprehensively and rigorously that the best route out of crisis will be found.

The conceptual crisis in the health world has not appeared overnight, nor will it be resolved dramatically. Developments occur slowly and infrequently, but significant changes are happening. In the British health service there has been progress towards increasing openness to innovation in both theory and practice. For over two hundred years in the Western nations professional health care has been associated almost exclusively with medicine and the medical establishment, but in recent years new trends and forces have emerged as challengers to the traditional order. Some of these pressures have been generated by the dissatisfaction and disquiet of people who have experienced the medical version of health care as 'outsiders', but many have occurred as a natural consequence of there being theoretical and practical problems that traditional medicine is badly equipped to tackle. Such forces inevitably pose a challenge to the very idea that medicine is and should be the single focus of health care.

It is possible to compare the crisis to a situation in which a ruling power finds it necessary to confront revolutionaries, but for the health service there need be no specific rebels—no one with an overt intention to question the establishment. This 'threat' is evolving as the discipline grows and matures. The members of the discipline have begun to ask searching questions about the rationale of a health service, about what a health service should truly be for, and about the relationship between ethics and health care. The conclusions that are dawning have massive implications for the whole organization and structure of health care.

Landmarks

There are a number of landmarks which announce a new era. These will come to be seen as signposts within a revolution in health care.

Among the most significant indicators that health work is in crisis are:

- The rise in the popularity of alternative methods of treating disease and illness. Several of these alternatives clash fundamentally with the traditional medical, reductionist theories of the nature of disease (West and Trevelyan 1985).
  (Note: reductionism is the theory that the fullest understanding of any object or event can be had only by reducing that object or event to its smallest constituent parts. Thus, reductionism asserts that an appreciation of molecular structure allows us to understand more about a piece of coal than the mere observation of it burning, and the understanding of the atomic structure of the coal creates yet deeper knowledge.)

- The increasing interest in the idea of 'holism' and 'holistic medicine'.

- The acknowledgement by some practising clinicians that it has become necessary for medicine to examine not only its most central tenets about how medical practice relates to morality, but also its fundamental beliefs about the nature and causes of disease, and the extent to which medical interventions can be effective at all (Greaves 1979).

- The recognition in medical education of the importance of ensuring meaningful and moral communication between doctors and patients. For example, instead of concentrating only on correct diagnosis and appropriate prescribing in general practice training, there is now in many medical schools strong emphasis on doctors concentrating on genuinely understanding patients' worries, on doctors being warm and approachable, on empathy, on dialogue, and on enabling patients to address their problem and condition for themselves. Although the manipulation of patients' behaviour 'for their own good' remains one possible rationale it is being challenged by a new philosophy, one which holds an important message about the ways in which people ought to be thought of and treated in society as a whole (see Metcalfe in Seedhouse and Cribb 1988).

- The appreciation, by members of the medical profession, of the fact that the role of medics working for health is relatively limited when compared to the role or potential role of politicians and environmentalists (WHO 1986).

- The impetus to include training and examinations in ethics for medical undergraduates (The Pond Report, Institute of Medical Ethics 1987).

- Movement towards improving communications between different sections of the NHS coupled with an examination of old hierarchies (The Cumberledge Report, DHSS 1986).

- The pressure from nurses to drag nursing courses away from the old idea of training in technique only towards the additional goal of providing nursing students with higher education in academic settings. Nurse education is still intended to produce skilled and competent nurses, but the plan is for the 'new nurse' to be a thoughtful nurse with the knowledge and experience to form her own judgements at work (United Kingdom Central Council for Nursing, Midwifery, and Health Visiting 1986).

- The acceptance of the medical establishment that it is both possible and desirable for nurses to be seen as practitioners in their own right (see Cleary in Seedhouse and Cribb 1988).

- The establishment of 'well-women' centres and associated 'health centres' in community settings (Gardner 1983).

- The growing emphasis on 'health promotion' as an endeavour which does not centre on medical practice and intervention.

- Ivan Illich's polemic against the counter-productivity of medicine and the mythology which surrounds the medical establishment—and the growth in the scrutiny of medicine by other academics and commentators spawned by 'Limits to Medicine'. The significance of Illich's contribution was, through careful research, his success in raising public awareness of the imperfections of medicine in practice, and of the emptiness of some of medicine's theoretical justifications for its practice.

- The continuing clarification of the range and significance of various ideas about the nature of health. This enterprise has taken place continually throughout history. The notion of health has always been and will continue to be contested by people with different points of view, politics, and imaginations. For instance, the decision to describe drug education and sex education as 'health education' is not based on any objective fact. People with different values might judge the misuse of drugs to be an issue for political education (if it is felt that the cause of the drug misuse can be traced directly to social policy and structure), and they might also judge that contraception and pregnancy should not be issues for medicine (and so come under the heading 'health education' via this route). And if drug education and sex education are to be described as issues for health education because sex and drugs (and presumably rock 'n roll) can cause disease, illness and injury, then why is general education, or do-it-yourself, not health education also?

Can any form of education or training be health education? On analysis it becomes clear that this is not so. It is possible to have a clear picture of the meanings of health and of the underlying unifying notion. Even without this comprehension, the facts that the arguments about the notion of 'health' persist, and that the task of defining health continues to be seen as important, reveal the extent to which the idea of 'health' has a great emotional impact, and how the way in which it is understood has implications not only for medical services, but for the organization and functioning of societies in general.

An Image is Changing

The business of providing health care solely through medicine is now under serious threat. The historical domination of health work by medicine can be understood in two ways. First, the domination can be said to have come about because of the high status and power that the medical profession possesses. Secondly, and more recently, the domination can be judged to have occurred as a result of the special knowledge required to make use of new technologies, and the associated continued emphasis on reductionism. But although health work still appears to be as dominated by medicine as it ever was, beneath the surface, beneath the strong residual image, significant intellectual developments are taking shape even though the majority of health workers may not yet be aware of it.

The analogy between the intellectual crisis in health care and the crisis associated with political revolutions is strong. As is the case with political and social upheavals, in the field of health care there are both traditionalists and pioneers. The traditionalists think it right to remain loyal to the old flag, they wish to stay as part of the old medical regime, and are happy to be, or be directed by, those who have supreme authority simply because they have had a medical training and have medical qualifications. The pioneers wish to open up a new era in health work (although they can only guess what its eventual shape will be) where issues such as unemployment, the distribution of wealth and power, social justice, the environment and education in general will all be legitimate targets for thought on, and action for, health (WHO 1986).

Thomas Kuhn and the Theory of Paradigms and Revolutions

It is not being claimed in this book that 'paradigms' actually exist. It is by no means clear what a paradigm actually is. The version offered below is one possible account, but there are others. Kuhn's theory of paradigms is valuable as a graphic analogy for the complex process of change that takes place over and between the different eras in the lives of fields of inquiry and practice. The theory of paradigms should be thought of as an aid to conceiving.

Thomas Kuhn, a philosopher and historian of science, has explored the idea of 'crisis of transition' in relation to the history of scientific research. Kuhn's theory is specifically concerned to describe and explain the attitudes and beliefs of groups of research scientists who work on shared projects. For the most part these scientists have common aims, accepted standards and procedures, and shared criteria of success for their endeavours. For most of the time, if not for their entire careers, these scientists will be engaged in what Kuhn calls 'normal science', where they will be trying to solve 'puzzles'—or technical difficulties—within the accepted tradition. Yet occasionally the scientists will be faced with a crisis which will cause them to question, at a deeper level, the most basic principles and assumptions of their research tradition. What was thought to be bedrock becomes quicksand, and all is uncertain. Events and results of experiments will be observed for which the current set of explanatory theories (the paradigm) is unable to account, and this will be accompanied by a growing collective perception that the existing way of viewing the whole project is fundamentally inadequate. This perception that 'there is something profoundly wrong about the theoretical framework in which we are working' can develop into a severe intellectual crisis which—after debate and the search for a more satisfactory direction, rationale, and set of beliefs- –can be resolved only by redefining the terms of the project. Such redefinition may be possible only when the most powerful researchers have become convinced of the validity of the new view.

A classic example of paradigm shift

The change in perspective that occurred when Newton's theory of mechanics was superseded by modern physics is often cited as a classic example of a scientific revolution or paradigm shift. Newton's mechanics provided a theoretical structure which endured and was applied fruitfully for over two centuries (Kuhn 1977). But as developments in technology both demanded and facilitated increasingly precise measurements and predictions Newtonian mechanics, was found to be not quite accurate enough. What happened was not an ever-developing increase in accuracy within the Newtonian tradition, instead Newton's mechanics was supplanted by an entirely different theoretical structure, one which explained the evidence in a way which differed radically from the account given by Newton. This was not a steady progression but a real upheaval, a real revolution in thinking. The implication for the understanding of the nature of science and the way in which it develops is immense, calling into question the 'common-sense' view that science is a steadily accumulating body of public knowledge about reality. From a study of other historical examples like this it seemed to Kuhn that this 'common-sense' view was not accurate, and that dramatic changes of direction can take place within research disciplines, even those that have achieved considerable practical success.

Newton's stature as a scientist and original thinker is unquestionable, yet his physical theories can no longer be built upon by modern physicists. Good research can be done which produces fundamentally mistaken theories. Consequently progress in science cannot be only a matter of building on existing work. Sometimes accepted theories and wisdoms have to be reassessed and rejected entirely or in part. This process happens in all research programmes, not just programmes in science.

Many philosophers of science do not agree with Kuhn, arguing that it is arbitrary and melodramatic to call a series of entirely explicable changes and developments a 'revolution'. Some critics point out that if the history of science is studied with care there are always strong strands of continuity and growth which are more fundamental than the apparently radical switches in perception (Lakatos and Musgrave 1970).

While it is clear that Kuhn's theory of paradigm change does not give a complete picture and explanation of developments in scientific research and theorizing, it is nevertheless enlightening to explore Kuhn's idea within the context of contemporary health care. There is much to learn from Kuhn's understanding of the history of science. The discussion which follows is over-simple, but it helps show how the idea of paradigm change can enable a fuller appreciation of developments in health work.

The Heart of the Crisis in Health Care

The basic idea of 'paradigm shift' can be illustrated as in Figure 1. This diagram represents the theory of paradigm change at its most simple. Paradigm X represents the old consensus, and Y its successor. The overlap represents the common ground remaining. In so far as the classic example is concerned, Newton and his contemporaries can be thought of as working in paradigm X. When it was discovered that Newtonian mechanics could not explain some astronomical observations paradigm X was thrown into crisis and a new paradigm assumed eventual dominance. In physics paradigm Y, which was to give birth to Relativity theory, the uncertainty principle, and quantum mechanics (Wolf 1981), was a radical departure from paradigm X. Many of the new basic assumptions contradicted Newtonian theory although some beliefs were still shared. For instance, the use of logic and mathematics, the demand that all theories should be tested as rigorously as possible, and the understanding of the terminology of the old paradigm, remained common (Lakatos and Musgrave 1970). In other words, even with this radical shift, the two spheres are not totally separate. Some philosophers of science maintain that the shift is not as neat or as simple as the Venn diagram illustration suggests, but that it usually makes more sense to think of the new paradigm as encompassing the old one, retaining the 'falsified knowledge' and mistaken beliefs, but finding this information of little or no relevance to future work (see Figure 2).

The abstract model of paradigm change can be carried into the world of health care as an aid to understanding. However, the model is not exactly appropriate since health care is concerned more with practice than research, and Kuhn's interest lay with scientific research. Nevertheless there is a partial analogy. As an example, perhaps the present health service might be thought of in the following way. This caricature is a gross simplification, and is included merely to illustrate the model of paradigm change. It is not always easy to distinguish the actual paradigm from the criticisms that are made of it, and already some other parts of paradigm X not listed below are elements that might become key features of a future paradigm.

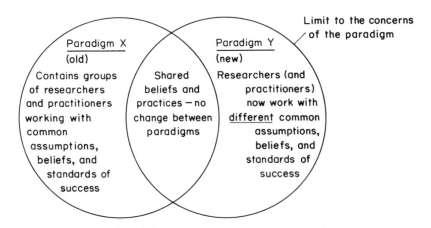

Figure 1   The paradigm shift in the abstract

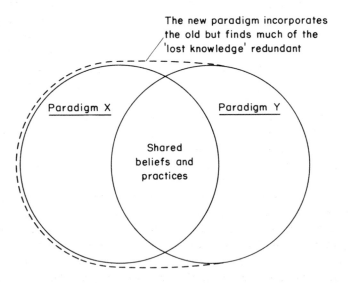

Figure 2   The new paradigm encompassing the old one

Paradigm X

Paradigm X contains the old school of health care where, for instance, health is thought to be nothing more than a state of a person who is not suffering from disease, illness, or infirmity; where the medical profession defines its own rationale and influence without consulting those it seeks to serve, where the central idea that informs 'medical education' is that as many 'facts' and technical skills as possible should be digested and crammed by students who become easily stressed and tired, and who soon come to see their 'education' only in instrumental terms—something to be 'got through' to become a doctor; where the idea of providing students, who daily will have to make crucial decisions about the lives and existences of other human beings, with a proper grounding in ethics is seen as pointless—or worse, seen as a threat; where technical decisions are made 'for the good of the patients' without the involvement of the patients; where patients are used to test the effect of drug treatments in controlled experiments without their knowledge; where patients are not permitted to see their medical records; where the health service is organized in strict hierarchical lines where everyone knows his or her place; where curing disease through clinical science is the primary motivation; and where the measures of success or failure of the care of patients are predominantly quantifiable and include severity of disease, deviation from measured norms, and life expectancy.

Paradigm Y

Paradigm Y contains (or is) the fruition of the developments, initiatives, and visions listed on pp. 4–5, plus a number of other practical improvements (see final chapter for examples). The vital difference between the paradigms is that paradigm Y is based on a different theoretical understanding of what work for health is about. Instead of the priorities of paradigm X the impetus of paradigm Y is the simple idea that people are of fundamental importance. Paradigm Y rests on a new analysis of what people are for—of what human existence is all about. In paradigm Y curing disease and illness and increasing the length of life remain important, but not as important as creating and increasing the autonomy of people who request or need health care, as distributing available resources according to need, as education, and as respecting people's choices even if they conflict with given advice (although there are limits to how far the choices ought to be respected—see pp. 131–2).

The manifestations of this enlightened rationale might include the overt acknowledgement by those in charge of the health service that health is more than the absence of disease, illness, and infirmity. This acknowledgement might be based on a clear and general understanding of the key factors of health. Part of such an account might involve the explanation that health, in its richest sense, is more to do with personal liberty than it is to do with personal fitness. The health service might be organized in a way which ensures that all its workers have a say in what happens to it; the users of the service might be allowed to see whatever has been written about them and be fully involved in all decisions that affect them. The task of enabling people to develop mentally, physically, and emotionally—creatively throughout their lives—might become a primary motivation (see Figure 3), thus necessitating a major restructuring of every health service (see final chapter).

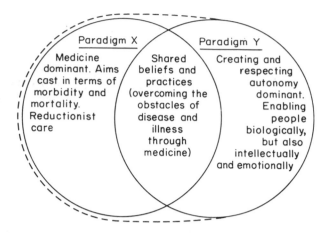

Figure 3   A possible paradigm shift for/in health care

A hidden crisis?

Paradigm Y in health care has not yet crystallized. The version of paradigm Y outlined in this book is put forward as a possibility, as something to be worked for.

The current turmoil has developed over several years and will calm only gradually. But some health workers do not accept this interpretation. Many people currently working for health will dismiss the initial argument of this book on the ground that the 'evidence' that health care is 'in crisis' is superficial. The counter-argument might state that there have been some changes of emphasis, and some secondary developments, such as holistic medicine, which complement the main body of medical work. But this slow evolution does not constitute an intellectual crisis, and clinical medicine rightly dominates health work.

However, it is important to reserve judgement until the full case has been made. The case is reinforced by a further discovery made by Kuhn. During his investigation into the history of scientific research Kuhn noticed that during the 'crisis period'—the time when two paradigms are competing for the ascendancy—only very few people recognize that the turmoil exists and that transition is happening. Some may suspect that a revolution is occurring but it is only with hindsight that the true extent of the crisis becomes apparent.

It is not surprising that so much escapes the attention of health workers who are committed to their particular tasks and specialisms. There is little time to stand back and reflect on changes that happen even within specific disciplines. The complexity of each discipline within health work makes detached assessment difficult. Standing back to take a broad view of the range of health disciplines can appear impossible to those involved in dealing daily within the many distressing obstacles that hinder and disable people they are devoted to helping. It is necessary to learn of disparate developments, pressures, and changes, to have at least a working knowledge of other workers' specialisms, and to enter into analysis complex enough to permit a comprehensive understanding of what is happening. For all of us working during the transition, as with political revolutions, it is only when the dust has settled that a complete picture can be seen.

The gestalt switch

Kuhn uses a further illustration to strengthen his argument. He claims that the change of perception and interpretation that happens when an individual notices that he is now working within a new paradigm can be likened to a 'gestalt-switch'. The idea of 'gestalt-switch' is one of many derived from the Gestalt school of psychology which developed at the start of the century. This school of thought criticized the Behaviourist account of perception which held that complex sensory events were nothing more than the sum of individual nervous impulses. The Gestalt school argued that some perceptual experiences show that a person's own contribution to what is seen cannot be ignored if a full explanation is to be given, and that sometimes the whole (i.e. the Gestalt) experience is more than the sum of sensory impulses. One illustrative example is that of the presentation of several photographs, each only slightly different from the one before, in rapid succession to give cinematographic motion. The Gestalt school pointed out that all the eye has received is a number of discrete still photographs, yet the subjective perception is one of motion. The conclusion has to be drawn that the brain adds to the sensations it receives from the outside world—human beings have a unique part to play in the creation of the realities which we experience (Ellis 1938).

The idea of the 'gestalt-switch' develops the theme. It is possible to see an arrangement of lines on paper in different ways. A picture might be seen as either a duck or a rabbit, for instance, and another picture as either a vase or two faces, according to what we think we are seeing (Figure 4). The point is that the theories we have about what we are observing help us to make sense of what we observe. Kuhn extrapolated this idea into the realm of science where if we hold one theory (for instance, that of Newtonian mechanics) we 'see' the evidence in one way, yet if we hold an alternative theory (for instance, the new theory of physics) we actually 'see' precisely the same evidence in a different way.

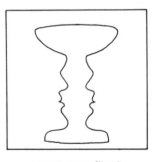
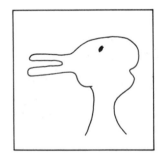

Vases or profiles?   A duck or a rabbit?

Figure 4   Examples of the gestalt-switch

It is possible to develop this line of thought even further, in a way that makes it directly relevant to health studies and health work. The theories that people hold about their everyday work, the subjective theoretical framework in which they operate, can affect their interpretations and understandings about what they do. The understanding that health workers have of their practice affects their performance and their attitude towards those they are caring for. It is crucial to make these interpretations as clear and overt as possible since a variety of subjective understandings exist. By highlighting the most moral understandings it will be possible to shape future developments to correspond with the richest sense of health. It will be possible to speed the formation of the new paradigm, and to ensure that it emerges with the most enlightened and egalitarian rationale.

Health Workers Can Create Future Change Through Present Practice

The degree to which paradigms are determinate and predictable is an open question. Perhaps events unfold according to some predetermined plan, perhaps human beings have no say at all in what happens to us. Speculations about the extent to which we have free will, or are merely pawns in some game. are intriguing but none can be verified conclusively (Kenny 1978).

Given this uncertainty it is wise to assume that human initiatives can affect the future, at least to some extent. And given this assumption it follows that the shape of the new paradigm is, to some degree, up to health workers. The paradigm is changing. It is up to health workers to ensure that the best features, those features that are truly part of the full sense of health, finally crystallize.

An illustration from science fiction

The significance of choosing one path rather than another, of opening the correct doors and leaving closed the remainder, has been demonstrated in a quaint short story, 'Opposite number', written by John Wyndham. The idea is that every 'instant' an atom of time splits. The two halves then continue upon different paths and meet different influences as they progress. And, like the pattern of radiating ribs of a fan, each half splits each instant too, *ad infinitum*.

The story of 'Opposite number' centres on a man and a woman. These characters—Peter and Jean—meet themselves! That is, when one particular 'atom of time' split, instantly there were not one but two couples—two Peters and two Jeans. Each of the couples had exactly the same history up until a crucial point in time when they began to follow different paths. One of the points that Wyndham appears to make is that the actual paths that develop are somehow dependent upon the personalities of the various Peters and Jeans, and upon the decisions they make.

One of the couples is a happy, married pair. The other Peter happens to meet this couple, who are able to explain the theory of 'splitting' to him. This other Peter had fallen out with the other Jean three years previously. It turns out that the paths of the couples diverted following a crucial conversation/argument, which through discussion the two Peters and Jeans are able to identify. One couple overcame possible conflict through the use of reason, in a friendly way, while for the other couple the argument ended their relationship.

Wyndham does not elaborate this point but the story could be read as arguing that people have great responsibility for what happens to themselves and others. Often what appears to be trivial turns out to have major consequences. Through our everyday actions we are responsible for creating one future rather than an indefinite number of other possible futures.

A parallel for health work

It is this emphasis on personal responsibility for creating the future—even in ways that appear insignificant—that is important. There is a major implication for health workers in Wyndham's story in that it is not only what they say about the future, but what they do now—in everyday practice—that will be instrumental in creating the future, in ensuring the crystallization of the new paradigm of richer health work.

As John Wyndham attempted to demonstrate in his science fiction story, we are *constantly* faced with a range of choices which will shape our destiny. We may have our paths limited by what we have done already, by our talents, our education, our circumstances, and the historical era in which we exist, but we always have a choice about what to do: what to believe, how to act towards others, and what to say. In very exceptional cases of limited choice there will still be alternatives open to us. For instance, at work we may have no choice but to teach a class of disinterested and unruly teenagers, but we still have significant options about how to deal with this, about how to treat the children, and about how to do justice to ourselves. And even where choice appears to be almost totally limited we can at least choose between doing and not doing a thing. We can create ourselves to some degree.

And just as we can create ourselves, through our actions we can create conditions in which other people are better placed to create more fulfilled versions of themselves. During the crisis, during the period of paradigm transition, it becomes even more vital for health workers not only to speak of 'positive health' and 'empowering' but also to act according to richer ideas than according to the tenets of the old, medically dominated paradigm. A person's actions are the acid test of his beliefs. It is not enough to believe, for instance, that individual autonomy should be a major priority for health work—and should sometimes be placed above that of a duty to prolong life—and yet to conform in practice to the latter principle. If the best new paradigm is to gain ascendancy over the dying one, in other words if the best of the alternatives is to be made into reality, then those health workers who believe in the principles of the new paradigm must ensure that they are true to themselves, and that their actions match their opinions.

Disease or Health?

The analogy of the 'gestalt-switch' can help to explain the issue at the heart of the paradigm transition in health work. It provides a powerful tool for illuminating a striking misperception that every partially enlightened health worker, or researcher into health issues, is experiencing during this crisis period. Gestalt-switch problems are not necessarily permanent or insoluble, they can be overcome. The way to break the 'gestalt-trap' is to display and explain both options simultaneously. This is not difficult in some cases (see Figure 4). Do you want to see either a duck or a rabbit, or do you want to be able to say, 'I see them both. Now I can make up my mind which I prefer'?

Clarification of meaning is crucial

The nature of practical work for health hinges ultimately upon the question of what health means. If 'work for health' is taken to mean only work to cure disease then the implications for practice will be substantially different from if 'work for health' is taken to mean 'liberating all human potential to the fullest degree'. In an earlier book, *Health: The Foundations of Achievement* (Seedhouse 1986), a number of different meanings and theories of health were introduced and discussed. Among these theories were the views that 'health is a state of complete physical, social and mental well-being, not merely the absence of disease, illness and infirmity'. This is the view of the World Health Organization. It is well-intentioned but not analysed with enough rigour. The 'fullest sense of health' proposed in *Health: The Foundations for Achievement* was intended to remain true to the intention of the WHO, but also to add real practical substance to it. Further theories discussed included the theory that health occurs when disease is absent; the theory that a person is healthy if she can perform her normal social function; and the theory that health is a strength, an ability to cope with or adapt to the problems that life throws in people's paths. Each of these theories has the merit of conforming to the overall sense of the notion of 'health', but these theories are not fully compatible with each other. They will not gel into a coherent whole without producing contradictions of meaning. For example, a person might have a disease (and so not conform to one possible meaning of 'health') and yet still be able to perform her normal social function (so conforming to an alternative meaning of 'health').

The analysis in the book reveals that the underlying sense that informs the various theories is that work for health is always designed to remove *obstacles* that lie in the path of biological, intellectual, emotional, and creative potentials latent in individuals. It was concluded, by drawing on this underlying sense, that 'health' is a far richer idea, an idea that relates to human flourishing in both mind and body, rather than a notion that is merely to do with the absence of disease. However this does not mean that focus on disease is not genuine health work. It is a significant part of work for health but not the whole story.

By drawing on this analysis it is possible to recognize the reality of the 'gestalt-trap' in the present crisis. Consider the title 'Health Promotion and Disease Prevention Officer'. The fact that two separate terms, 'health promotion' and 'disease prevention' are used implies either that they have different meanings or else that one or the other is merely superfluous. It has been shown that 'health promotion' does have a range of meanings which differ in varying degree from 'disease prevention'. By reflecting on the meanings of the two terms it is possible to highlight the fact that there is a tension, as yet perceived only dimly by many health workers, between the idea that health is dynamically yet inextricably linked only to illness, and the emerging view that health is truly to do with the extent to which a person is equipped to live a life in which she can work to fulfil the potentials she has. Much of the present confusion and ambiguity in health studies and work for health have come about because this major distinction is not perceived to be a distinction at all. Forward-looking authors writing about health issues frequently introduce rather nebulous ideas such as 'positive health' and 'well-being' as one way of indicating that health is something more than the absence of illness and not one side of a see-saw with illness the exact counter-balance. But then, as happens with the 'gestalt-switch', having glimpsed another perspective momentarily—a duck rather than a rabbit—they slip back into the old habit of discussing *only* how to decrease disease and illness. Often, when their works are studied with knowledge of the other side of the 'gestalt-switch' in health care, it is apparent that these writers have thought to themselves that health means something such as 'being fulfilled as a person', or 'gaining autonomous control over one's life and environment'. Seen from this perspective powerful and complex notions of freedom, justice, and equality become at least as important as those of disease and illness.

Often the question of whether or not a person is diseased or ill need never be part— or at least only a small part—of any thinking about the state of a person's health. Health writers and workers who are caught in the present 'gestalt-trap' can realize briefly that health is to do with personal fulfilment, but then they hit a daunting mental block. As soon as they begin to consider how this fulfilment can be made concrete, how what is potential can become actual, they fall back under the spell of medicine, hurtled backwards as if attached to a piece of elastic that has been stretched as far as it can go. The basic problem is that health is still popularly thought of from a point of reference which begins with disease, rather than as a quality in its own right.

Health education staff, employed by the British health service, provide a clear example of the gestalt trauma. Thoughtful health educators *say* that health is more than the absence of disease and illness, but their official work is entirely directed at preventing disease and illness. Having experienced a fleeting insight into the fullest sense of health the very next thought of the ensnared health educator is always something like, 'How can I persuade this person to adopt the kind of habits which will make him less prone to becoming ill?' Certainly, if a health educator can achieve this particular goal then she stands a good chance of improving that person's quality of life (for instance, if the person who is the target of the persuasion avoids a stroke as a result then this is almost certainly a good thing). The problem is that constant emphasis on ameliorating disease and illness in the name of health perpetuates a central mistake—that is, the continuation of the unreflective assumption that preventive and curative medicine is the best means of helping an adult person to become more fulfilled, to become more of what she could be. Yet it is not. Health is not only a matter for medicine and can be created and improved in numerous ways in which medicine has no brief.

Summary

The argument advanced so far has been this:

1. A range of forces can be identified that are symptomatic of an intellectual crisis in the world of health care. Because of the confusion generated by this crisis it is likely that there are other forces for change which will become apparent only in the new era. It is immaterial whether or not paradigms have any real existence. All that needs to be acknowledged is that change for the better is possible.
2. Although the time scale over which the paradigm shift will occur cannot be predicted, it is inevitable that a new framework for health care will eventually crystallize. It is likely that this new framework will be based on ideas and principles drawn from a richer view of health than is currently popular.
3. Although certain forces can be pointed out that seem to compel the paradigm shift to occur, it is not possible to predict the final shape of the new paradigm. The future of health care might take on a variety of alternative shapes.
4. It falls to health workers to ensure that the best alternative becomes a reality, and much depends upon what present health workers think and how they act.

The Next Challenge

The tasks for health workers are these:

1. To be clear about the range of principles of health care that exist.
2. To expose the principles that must inform the *richest* possible work for health.
3. To put these principles into practice during the period of crisis. In other words, to act according to these principles as soon as possible.
4. To ensure that the new paradigm which must form is the best theoretical framework possible.

But how is all this to be done? How can such a mammoth task be attempted coherently? How can a new set of principles be agreed upon by people with divergent interests? How can the ambition to create a new era of health work be achieved without being destroyed at birth by party political arguments? How can the principles of the new paradigm be given their correct importance—how can they be explained so that they assume their true significance above the directly pragmatic issues of administration, staffing, resource allocation, and territory battles?

An Answer

The answer is at once stunningly simple and frustratingly complex. It lies in the fact that there is an ultimate and fundamental link between the idea of *health* and the idea of *morality*. This link has not, up to now, been noticed to anything like its fullest extent. Health work is moral work. Consequently, by making clear the range and importance of the moral content of health work, by bringing what already exists to the fore in its proper focus, it will be possible to bring about the most desirable form of the new paradigm. Simply, ethics is the key to the formation of the new era of health work.

Chapter Two
Ethics is the Key

After an introductory chapter that has drawn attention to the existence of a conceptual crisis in the health world, to changes of practice that reflect this conceptual crisis, and to the idea of paradigms and gestalt-switches, it might come as a surprise that this book is not to be devoted explicitly to these topics. Instead the bulk of the analysis is given over to a studied consideration of the idea and application of ethics. And the entire theory presented and built up throughout this account of health work rests on a particular view of the nature of ethics.

Yet there are those who regard ethics as at a best a secondary issue for health work and medical work, and some economists believe that ethical issues are not relevant to health care at all. However, it will become clear, as this inquiry blossoms, that far from ethics being of peripheral interest in health work, ethics is the key which can release thoughtful health workers from their present gestalt limbo. The key to the door out of crisis is ethics. Creating health creates morality. *Work for health is a moral endeavour*. This is the slogan of the new paradigm.

'Work for Health is a Moral Endeavour'

Why a slogan, and what does it mean?

Slogans on their own are empty. Without the support of argument and reason they are nothing more than battle cries. This slogan is supported by the weight of reason contained in this book. It should not be used without an understanding of the arguments which lie behind it. But if the arguments are understood then the slogan can serve as a focus for attention, a constant reminder of the reason for working for health, and a starting point for explanation to others who do not yet understand how the future of health care might be.

A query

But what does the slogan mean? How, it might be asked, is work for health a *moral* endeavour? Certainly health is desirable, according to common sense to be healthy is surely a good thing, but this is not related to morality. 'Being moral' is an idea that is related to *specific* dilemmas and issues, where it is important to distinguish clearly between good and bad and right and wrong. Surely it is a disastrous confusion to mistake being healthy for goodness, and somehow associating being unhealthy with doing or being wrong?

A response

This book argues that work for health in its richest sense is equivalent to work for morality in its richest sense. Health work is moral work. Consequently, all health work interventions can be more or less moral, and so more or less in accord with the richest sense of health. Morality should not be thought of as being clear-cut. It is better to imagine that morality has an indefinite number of degrees, on a continuum running from the immoral to the highest degree of morality. The precise nature of the various degrees, and their rankings, is an open question.

It would be a disastrous confusion to associate the idea of morality and health in the way described by the query. This is a form of 'victim-blaming', a phenomenon where people are held to be to blame for illnesses they happen to be suffering from, when the causes of these illnesses are not within their control. This is not what is intended. Nor is the intention of this book to argue that the moral element of health work enters the picture only when specific dilemmas are clearly apparent. Ethics is not only of relevance when specific issues arise, such as 'Should life support machines ever be switched off?' or 'Is it right to prescribe contraceptives to a fifteen year old girl against the wishes of her parents?' or 'Should all mentally sub-normal children be sterilized?' Instead, the view of this book is that ethics permeates all aspects of health work. This must be so because on reflection it becomes clear that it is simply not possible to understand the nature of health work properly without understanding the nature of ethics.

What is Ethics?

Ethics can be complex

Introductory remarks   (Note: in this book no distinction is made between 'ethics' and 'morality'. All variations of the words can be used interchangeably.)

'Ethical' and 'moral' are words whose significance and meaning enter into all areas of human thought and action. Ethics is concerned with how men and women ought to live their lives. The range of issues that have implications for ethics is immense and varied. As a means of clarification this diversity can be dissected into different compartments. Each compartment will inevitably overlap with others in places. This process of separation can become complicated and intricate. Ethics can be divided into types. Some of these types contain major theories which can be divided further (see Chapter 7). However, it is possible and important to show, by a very basic separation, that it is mistaken to think of ethics as a single coherent body of knowledge and opinion about what is right and what is wrong. The issue is far more complicated than this. This introductory separation is given here in order to prepare health workers to see the complexity, and to be able to ask the most appropriate questions about their work.

A distinction   We have all experienced discussions on moral issues. Debates about right and wrong, about what is moral behaviour and what is immoral, are very common. These discussions happen daily: at work, over shop counters, in public houses, on trains, at bus stops—everywhere where people are interested and concerned enough to discuss issues affecting human life and relationships. Beliefs are expressed about certain principles which we argue should be followed by other people, and which we might also set as standards of personal behaviour. These everyday ethical reflections and judgements are important, but they are usually not the result of thorough analysis. Sometimes people advocate principles that are inconsistent. This inconsistency might be acceptable at the level of casual debate and conversation—everyday ethics—but for another type of ethics—technical ethics—inconsistencies must be avoided at all costs.

Everyday ethics

The term 'everyday ethics' is not intended to be derogatory. Everyday ethics can often be more sincere and genuine than any other variety of ethics. The term 'everyday ethics' is used merely to indicate a difference in kind between more intuitive and spontaneous reactions to life situations and dilemmas, and those grounded in more abstract theory and principles, and formed according to logic and analytic consistency. The everyday ethics of different people can vary immensely, both in content and in consistency.

One example of everyday ethics A disadvantage with everyday ethics is that, since little attention is paid to overall consistency or to a guiding rationale, decisions that are made can be taken purely according to 'the moment', purely according to the context and the emotional state of the person at that time. Different contexts might give rise to different, even contradictory, ethical intuitions. Consider this example of everyday ethics, one conceivable basic grounding for intuition.

Dependent upon context this example of a 'system' of everyday ethics uses the following simple principles, possibly in varying forms, as a framework for a response to life issues and dilemmas: 'sex before marriage is wrong', 'it is wrong to be underhand and deceitful at work', 'people who look after number one should be respected', 'you should always respect the wishes of other people', 'you should take only what a job is worth', 'adultery is acceptable so long as the adulterers are happy and no one gets hurt'. This is one possible framework drawn from an indefinite number of others. If all the possible frameworks of all everyday ethics were to be incorporated into a grand theory then the contradictions and conflicts contained within would be quite impossible to resolve. Even with the simple example of an everyday ethics given above there are many contexts which call the consistency of the basic framework into question.

Each dictum refers to different, or slightly different, subject areas. Each dictum might be justifiable in certain contexts. For example, respecting the wishes of other people rather than always being authoritarian might produce the most favourable outcome for all concerned in certain contexts (perhaps in many doctor–patient relationships). Also, the dictums 'people who look after number one should be respected' and 'it is wrong to be underhand and deceitful at work' might, taken in combination, produce the most favourable outcome. For instance, there could be spin-off benefits for others from enterprising self-interest, and especially if such enterprise is undertaken openly and without deceit. But there are other contexts where such a combination of dictums is not consistent or compatible, and this seriously undermines the 'grounding framework' of this, and similar, everyday ethics. Perhaps the self-interested man understands the best way of 'looking after number one' to be to embezzle his employer's profits (so being deceitful and underhand at work). In this context the rather *ad hoc* grounding for intuitive response is shown to be contradictory. It seems that if a consistent ethical position is desired then something more than *ad hoc* frameworks and instant intuitions are needed. It has been argued that technical ethics, which is inspired by a more rigorous understanding, can offer this extra element.

Technical ethics

'Technical ethics' sets out to avoid the inconsistencies of 'everyday ethics', although some types of technical ethics have to pay a different price—they have to sacrifice flexibility and the achievement of the highest possible degree of morality for the sake of consistency.

It is the job of moral philosophers to devise and refine technical ethical theory. 'Technical ethics' refers to a number of theories that have been analysed and thought through carefully to try to ensure that contradictions raised by context do not occur. The aim of a moral philosopher is to design a theory that is internally coherent, which contains principles and notions that are consistent and complement each other, and which will enable a person to 'act morally' (at least in so far as the particular technical ethical theory is concerned) whatever the situation in life which confronts him.

Ethics and the Tip of the Iceberg

Technical ethics can be subdivided into a range of aspects. Before some of these are indicated it is necessary to make another clarification.

A further distinction

A distinction can be made between *dramatic* or *specific* ethics, *persisting* ethics, and ethics in a *general sense*. This distinction is not clear-cut or fully watertight, but it helps explain how issues which do not appear to be dilemmas can, nevertheless, be seen to be ethical issues.

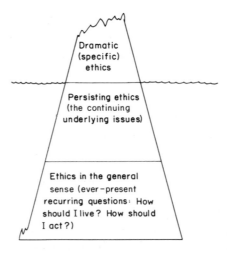

Figure 5 Ethics and the tip of the iceberg—a broad distinction between different types of ethics (not final or watertight)

This distinction can be thought of as a division between various parts of an iceberg. It is well known amongst those who have failed to think up a less clichéd image that only the tips of icebergs are visible above the water (see Figure 5).

Specific or dramatic ethics   'Specific ethics' refers to deliberation about the most moral course of action to take when one is presented with a specific dilemma, a dilemma that seems to stand self-contained, in isolation from other personal or work issues. Ethics in the specific sense takes place when one is confronted with a hard choice. For instance, the choice might be whether to switch off a life support machine in order to be able to transplant a variety of organs to three waiting recipients, all of whom stand a good chance of further fulfilling life, or whether to keep the machine on because of the slim possibility that the body might regain consciousness.

In a dilemma such as this a clear decision has to be made. Dependent on the decision certain consequences will follow with a high probability. The pros and cons, both morally and practically, are reasonably clear. All that is required further is the courage to take one course of action or the other—to say, specifically, yes or no.

'Dramatic ethics' is concerned with 'tragic choices', with decisions where one must fall into one camp or the other—where 'sitting on the fence' is not possible. Dramatic ethics features frequently in television documentaries, especially on Sunday evenings. Examples of dramatic ethics might include the presentation of debates about whether or not it is right to sterilize sexually aware Down's syndrome children, or whether it is right for women to sign contracts to be surrogate mothers, effectively agreeing to sell their child, or the morality of abortion, or whether it is right to manufacture and sell arms to other countries. This focus by the various media on dramatic ethics has led to the common perception that such 'hot spots' are all that there is to ethics.

This is ethics at the tip of the iceberg.

Persisting ethics   As a result of this exposure, 'persisting ethics' has been underplayed. Included in this category are the continuing issues which constantly underlie the dramatic cases which come into focus from time to time. For example, underlying the question of whether or not abortion should be a legal right are constant and more fundamental questions concerning, for instance, what it is to be a person or potential person, and the degree of control that a woman ought to have over the treatment of her body.

Ethics in a general sense   Ethics in a general sense refers, at its simplest, to frequent deliberation—both abstractly and concretely—about how best to conduct one's life. The person who deliberates in a general sense of ethics realizes that moral questions do not occur only occasionally, but that all thought and all action can and should produce moral reflection in individuals. It might not, for example, be instantly obvious that a decision about whether or not to pass the salt on request to a friend at a dinner table, or whether or not continue sitting in an armchair doing nothing, have a relevance to morality, but they do in this general sense.

The point is that whatever one does, either to oneself or to another person, does not have to be done. There are always alternative courses of action possible. And these alternatives can have different consequences. Dependent upon what one chooses to do, one can encourage or enhance one's own or another's existence to different degrees.

To take the examples: if you are asked to pass the salt at dinner you can do this gladly or begrudgingly—perhaps causing the other person to feel more or less at ease. The consequence of feeling more at ease might be that he will enjoy his meal more, and perhaps be more prepared to make interesting conversation than he otherwise would. Or, if you know something about nutrition and heart disease you might decide to inform your friend of the possible consequences of excessive consumption of salt—you might tell him this casually, or jokingly, or seriously; you might even scare him and cause him to feel guilty or stressed about his past habits.

And if you are sitting in an armchair you might be doing something else. There is no compulsion on a person to do something else if that is what he chooses (many people have defended Dennis in discussions (see Seedhouse 1986, p.4)—although Dennis has remained unmoved by this show of support). It has been suggested that Dennis has every right to sit in an armchair all the time, if this is what he wishes. It has been pointed out that it is ridiculous to suggest that everyone should feel guilty about relaxing in armchairs. But the central point does not concern Dennis's civil rights, nor does it concern guilt (clearly people need to relax). The inescapable fact is that other things are possible. By remaining in the armchair (say you just happen to have woken up in the armchair and you simply continue to do nothing) you are doing little or nothing to create more of the possibilities open to yourself, and you are doing nothing to enable other people in any way. It may not be the depth of immorality to remain in an armchair simply because everyone has got to be somewhere, but neither is it the height of morality. You could be doing more.

Even sitting in an armchair is a moral question.

The distinction between the specific and the general breaks down when one sees the importance and implications of the general sense of ethics. But the distinction, although artificial, is nevertheless enlightening since it begins to make clearer the way in which work for health must be seen as a moral endeavour.

An illustration of the distinction   The conflict in 1982 between Great Britain and Argentina over the Falkland Islands (or Malvinas) gives an especially clear picture of the 'tip of the iceberg' phenomenon. The conflict flared quickly and was soon over. It focused intense interest in some quarters on certain specific or dramatic ethical issues. For instance, there was widespread discussion about the morality of killing hundreds of people over a relatively barren and sparsely populated island; about whether the principle of 'sovereignty' should take precedence over the principle of 'common humanity'; about whether Britain had a clear and certain *duty* to protect her citizens wherever they might be; and about whether lying and secrecy (by government in 'communication' with the general public) was ethically correct, even in time of war.

Although most of these dramatic ethical issues are no longer in the limelight the questions remain. And lying below these questions, at the next level below sea-level, are persisting ethical questions which existed before, during, and after the Falklands conflict. These questions are at least as important as the dramatic issues even though they are not so immediately apparent as the dramatic issues. For example, these persisting moral issues include the questions: Is it moral to maintain such a large army in peace time when the social and environmental conditions of millions of people in Britain are self-evidently poor and debilitating? Should the public have access to more information about the workings of the military? Should people have the right to refuse to pay taxation to maintain armed forces if they are pacifists? Should governments elected by a minority of people in the country have the right to call upon people to go to war?

At the base of the iceberg lies the area of ethics in the general sense. This form of ethics actually permeates the whole iceberg. For instance, when the focus is on ethics in the general sense a person might ask, 'What can I do about the dramatic and persisting issues?' 'Should I campaign to put over my point of view?' 'Should I distort evidence to persuade people of my position?' 'If I am with a group of relative strangers, perhaps in a pub after a few drinks, all of whom vehemently support a position to which I am strongly oppopsed, should I explain what I believe or should I let it pass?' Such questions are no less hard to answer than those raised in any other part of the iceberg.

Aspects of Technical Ethics

Now that certain illustrative distinctions have been made it is appropriate to present three aspects of 'technical ethics' in order to provide the student of health care ethics with an initial bearing, with some reasonably solid ground on which to stand.

All the following aspects encompass the complete iceberg. Each relates in part to ethics in the 'dramatic', the 'persisting', and the 'general' senses.

1. Moral philosophy as a quest to understand 'the good'

One major branch of technical ethics is not directed towards a means of confronting and solving immediate dilemmas and issues, although this can nevertheless be a consequence of the enterprise. This branch of moral philosophy seeks to understand the nature of 'goodness' itself. It is devoted to uncovering the essential features of what is truly right and what is truly wrong. It is argued that only by first understanding what 'goodness' means can those who wish to be good begin to attempt to be good.

The technicalities of this division of moral philosophy are not discussed in any detail. However, certain key features do require clarification.

A brief clarification of meaning   It is possible to become so preoccupied with questions of meaning that it is only meaning—and nothing else—that is seen as the problem. Two points need to be restated: first, it is crucial, in any serious inquiry, that the meanings of the key terms are clarified as far as possible; but secondly, it must not be thought that merely by clarifying the meanings of words real problems in the real world can be solved. The clarification of meaning is an essential part of inquiry into ethics, but it is only a part.

Good   It is important to emphasize that there is more than one sense of the word 'good'. This is apparent after a moment's reflection. It is possible to distinguish at least three separate senses of the word 'good':

(a) 'Good' as a description of objects that are useful, instrumental, or functional   For example, using this sense of 'good' people talk of a 'good clock' or a 'good motor car'. 'Good' in this sense appears to be ethically neutral, at least when the word is used only as a description. If the question is asked 'What is this good car being used for?' then

there is moral content. For example, the car might be being used by a volunteer to transport disabled people, or it might be a getaway car for armed robbers.

(b) 'Good' as a description of things that are pleasing or enjoyable in themselves   For example, using this sense of the word it is possible to describe an aesthetically pleasing painting, or a productive garden, as good. Again, 'good' in this sense appears to be ethically neutral because there are no direct moral implications associated with its use.

(c) 'Good' as a description of the specifically moral   When the word 'good' is used in this sense it is used to describe human activity, usually human activity that affects other people and not only the actor. The word good is applied not to things like clocks or gardens, but to people and their actions—to what we do or leave undone. This use of the word good has close connections with other 'moral words' such as 'ought', 'right', 'just', and 'duty'. For instance, it can be argued that a person ought to do what is good. Naturally each of these words requires detailed analysis as well as study in specific contexts.

2. Moral philosophy based on either consequences or duties

A central controversy in moral philosophy stems from the possibility of thinking of ethics in two ways that are apparently very different: between basing decisions about how to act on the assessment of the likely consequences or outcomes of actions, and basing decisions on beliefs about certain duties taken to be fundamental to the very idea of morality.

As an introduction consider these traditional examples:

Consequences   One theory in technical ethics is known as 'utilitarianism'. Utilitarians assess the worth or morality of what people do by looking either at the actual results (and so judging morality in retrospect) or by calculating the likely future outcomes of actions. For utilitarians the best actions, the most moral actions, are those which produce the greatest happiness or pleasure for mankind as a whole—those which produce the most favourable balance of good over evil in the world. So the worth of any action—whether a small kindness to another person, or a decision to declare war on another nation—is considered to be moral or not dependent on whether the outcome is a balance of human pleasure over human misery or not.

A slightly different theory of technical ethics is known as 'consequentialism'. Consequentialists also assess the worth of actions in terms of the results of the actions but they do not only consider the result in terms of pleasure or happiness. The particular 'good' is stated beforehand by the consequentialist, as part of the technical theory. Perhaps a 'decrease in disease levels' or an 'increase in higher educational opportunities' will be stated to be, and justified as, the 'good' or the most moral outcomes possible, even though neither is guaranteed to produce more happiness. So, for those moral philosophers who are consequentialists the outcomes will not be judged in terms of a balance of pleasure and happiness over misery, pain, and unhappiness, but in terms of a particular balance of good over evil which will have been specified beforehand by the moral philosopher.

Duties   Another version of technical ethics is known as 'deontology'. The theory is that what matters most is not the result but the fact that a person acted according to a perceived duty, and intended that some good should come about. For example, a moral philosopher who advocates deontology might argue that certain principles, perhaps truth-telling and promise-keeping, are fundamental to morality and that, to be moral, a person has a moral duty always to abide by these principles—whatever the consequences. Even if the outcome of telling the truth in a certain situation produces more misery than happiness, to tell the truth, to abide by preconceived moral duty is the right and honest way to act. Some deontologists do not consider the calculations of consequentialists to be moral reasoning at all. A feature central to deontology is the idea of integrity, that all decisions should be made genuinely by referring to honest principles rather than based on expedient calculation. The belief is that people do not count only as units to be measured and balanced, but that each human being is vastly important in herself, and that the mark of her moral stature is the integrity with which she abides by certain rules of conduct.

3. Moral philosophy as a process of deliberation

This type of technical ethics is different from the other types identified since moral philosophy as a process of deliberation makes no ultimate plea to duties or rules or past and future consequences. This type of moral philosophy is the version developed and espoused in this book. It is closer to the Aristotelian view of ethics than to any other type of ethics. This type of technical ethics can be split into two parts: *the process* of deliberation itself, and *the goal* which the deliberation is intended to achieve.

The process is not a blind or chance procedure. The depth of the reasoning depends upon the thinker having a grasp of a number of principles and methods, and also a personal sense of balance and maturity. The process can be enhanced by offering and clarifying guidelines on procedure, on ways of deliberation.

The aim of the deliberation process advocated in this book is concerned with the most fundamental form of morality possible. *The goal* is human flourishing. The idea is that the most moral form of endeavour is one which aims at producing more of what human beings are for, more enhancing human potential. All actions, if they are to express some degree of morality, should aim to create more of what human beings have the potential to be. The nature of this goal can be indicated, very simplistically for now, in this way. It is contained in the very nature of an acorn that it can become an oak tree. In order for the acorn to achieve this potential it must go through a number of stages of development successfully, the environmental conditions must be conducive to its proper development, and no serious obstacles must impede its growth (for the acorn and the potential oak these obstacles might include lumberjacks, drought, fires, diseases, locusts, or town planners). In a like but vastly more complicated and unpredictable way, it is in the nature of a day old child to become a uniquely fulfilled adult dependent upon personal and external conditions.

So the essence of this type of ethics is personal deliberation about the best ways in which to create more of what might be in oneself and others, in specific cases and throughout life generally. This version of moral reasoning is difficult to grasp if one believes that being ethical is a question of following specific rules and codes of conduct, or of always acting according to a specific view of what is right and wrong. However, as Aristotle recognized, it is the most fundamental form of moral reasoning.

Aristotle believed that deliberation is the essence of ethics. There has to be a process of deliberation in every case where conclusions have to be reached about the worth of human activity. Aristotle divided knowledge into three different disciplines: theoretical, practical, and productive (Aristotle 1976). The majority of his works were concerned with 'natural science'—where 'natural and regular laws' apply. This category falls under the heading 'theoretical'. According to Aristotle, under this heading there is no need for deliberation because this is the realm of fact, of mathematical law, and of predictable physical cause and effect. But ethics is essentially different. It does not have the certainty of 'natural science'. There is an indefinite—perhaps even infinite—variety of human circumstances and situations. and there can be no universal laws or sets of principles than can be applied to every situation. Whatever 'rule' is invented in moral philosophy, sooner or later a situation will occur in which it will be better to break the rule in order to create a better human potential. And because of this it is far better—far more moral—to enhance human judgement in the uncertain field of human action and interaction, rather than to instil imperfect sets of rules in people as if these rules are inviolable commandments. Rules and principles are useful to the deliberation process, but subjective judgement in context is ultimate.

Ethics and Health Workers

Many health workers have not, until now, had the opportunity to appreciate the enlightening distinctions that can be made within moral philosophy. Many health workers are able to see only the tip of the iceberg, yet it is only by discovering the entire iceberg that health workers can be instrumental in ensuring the emergence of the best form for the new paradigm. Health workers should not be blamed for this because:

1. With few exceptions health workers receive no formal training in ethics, even though their daily work involves direct and often crucial intervention in other people's lives.
2. Health workers usually have an urgent practical job to do which allows them little time to pause for thought. Currently there are no facilities within the NHS to permit classes and discussion groups to provide health workers with the opportunity to reflect on the issues, and so become more proficient in ethical deliberation and action.
3. Many books on ethics speak in a language and a manner which most health workers find alien (examples of such books can be found on library shelves between the Dewey classifications 170–174 or Library of Congress reference BJ). If examples are given in these books to illustrate moral theory they are frequently artificial and hypothetical. Such works often attempt to solve esoteric technical problems. These are genuine problems but can seem to be unrelated to everyday affairs.

Summary

In Chapter One it was argued that there is an intellectual crisis in health care. The form of health care that emerges in the future depends upon which theories of health come to dominate, and upon the ways in which present health workers act in their interventions in the lives of their clients. It was argued that the most desirable future—the best new paradigm—could be created if health workers understood better the nature of ethics, and if they recognized the implications of the slogan 'work for health is a moral endeavour'.

In this chapter the following points and clarifications have been made.

1. Work for health is a moral endeavour because work for health can release more or less of the potential of individuals. Roughly, the more enhancing potentials that are liberated the higher the degree of morality there has been in an intervention.
2. Ethics is a complex discipline. Moral philosophy is not merely a means of deciding between clear-cut rights and wrongs.
3. Enlightening distinctions can be made between 'everyday ethics' and 'technical ethics', and between dramatic/specific ethics, persisting ethics, and ethics in the general sense.
4. Technical ethics can be divided into different aspects. Ethics as deliberation is the aspect highlighted in this book since (a) it involves both process and aim, (b) it is closely associated with the idea of ethics in the general sense, and (c) it indicates acutely the way in which health work can be perceived as a moral endeavour.

Chapter Three
Uncovering the Basic Questions

> It appears to me that in Ethics as in all other philosophical studies, the difficulties and disagreements, of which its history are full, are mainly due to a very simple cause: namely to the attempt to answer questions, without firstly discovering precisely what question it is which you desire to answer. (Moore 1903, p. vii)

The question 'What is ethics?' has been debated for millennia. The safest answer to it so far is that ethics is not one body of thought but a range of different theories, related in some way that it is not easy to be clear about! This inquiry has other aims than to become entirely stuck on the question of the nature of ethics.

Instead the concern is this: because ethics is a range of different theories and beliefs, it is essential to be clear about which form is most relevant to the current inquiry. And the best means of discovering this is to be clear about the sorts of questions that are being asked, and, if possible, to identify a single key question which will act as a focus for the whole inquiry.

What is the Central Question for Health Work?

What question more than any other can be instrumental in forming the new paradigm? The central question in health work can be uncovered through an appreciation of the fullest sense of both 'health' and 'ethics'. Health work in its fullest sense is work aimed at preventing or eliminating obstacles that might or do stand in the way of individuals' biological and chosen potentials, so long as the achievement of these potentials causes no intentional harm to other human beings. And just as this is the true nature of work for health so it is the true nature of a moral endeavour, in the sense of ethics as a general process of deliberation.

What is the point of mending a broken leg? What is the point of helping a person overcome some emotional trauma through counselling? What is the point of trying to cure cancer? What is the point of attempting to enable a cancer sufferer to come to terms with his illness, and to accept the new limitations of his existence? *The point is to enable each person to achieve more of whatever potential they have to enhance their own lives and the lives of other people.*

A Vital Link

A fundamental link between health work and morality is this. Whatever the meaning that can be given to 'health', work for health is bound to involve some *intervention* in the life of oneself or of other people. That it is possible to intervene in lives—either for better or for worse—is the key to the importance of morality. Moral philosophers and others are concerned about human thought and action in so far as this thought and action has implications for that individual and other people who share the world. Whatever we choose to do we could have chosen to do otherwise. It follows that whatever sort of intervention we make we could also have intervened otherwise—or not at all.

Now in work for health a whole range of types of intervention are possible—all of which naturally have moral implications because interventions are precisely the subject matter of morality. For instance, consider the simple example of setting and mending a broken wrist (any health intervention example would serve equally well as an illustration).

Two scenarios

1. The first scenario   A young man has been playing football and, during a hopelessly optimistic attempt at an overhead kick, has landed awkwardly and has broken his left wrist. He does not know that he has a broken bone but is in great pain and so visits the casualty department. On reporting to reception he is told in an unfriendly way to sit and wait his turn. He asks how long he will have to wait, but the receptionist tells him that she has no idea. He then eats a packetful of boiled sweets. Three quarters of an hour later he is approached by a nurse who takes him to a doctor. The doctor mumbles at the young man and sends him to X-ray. The young man asks whether the bone is broken, and whether he need be in such pain, but the doctor shrugs and tells him not to be a baby. The X-ray shows that the bone is broken and needs to be reset. A nurse then arrives and asks the young man whether he has eaten anything during the last 24 hours, in order to see whether or not it will be safe to administer a general anaesthetic. The young man says that all he has eaten is a bagful of boiled sweets; the nurse says that she is sorry but all she can do is to administer a local anaesthetic.

The anaesthetic is administered and the young man is told to wait fifteen minutes for the pain to stop. But it persists. The young man tells the doctor this as he is about to take him into the side room to set the wrist. The doctor is surprised but reluctantly agrees to wait a further fifteen minutes. Still the pain persists and the young man is by now becoming very anguished and frightened. He tells the doctor that he is still in as much pain as ever but the doctor does not believe him and, ignoring his protests, begins to set the wrist. This causes the young man excruciating agony. He screams involuntarily and is held down by three nurses until the doctor has done his work. After further pain and screams the doctor is satisfied and, without a word to the young man—of either apology or explanation—the doctor leaves and a plaster cast is placed on the wrist by a surly technician. An appointment is made for the young man to return in two days' time to check that the broken bone is still in place. He is given advice to take paracetamol for the pain and to rest. Nothing else.

2. An alternative   The same young man has been playing football and, during the same ludicrous execution of an 'overhead kick', has broken his left wrist. He visits the casualty department. On reporting to reception he is treated with kindness and with sympathy. The receptionist, noting that the young man appears to be suffering a degree of shock (from the result of his injury rather than from any surprise at having performed so miserably), gives him a cup of tea from a dispenser behind her desk and tells him to sit and wait for the nurse who will attend him as soon as she has seen patients who arrived before him—this will probably be in half an hour or so. The receptionist asks the young man whether he has eaten for the last 24 hours (it is now around lunch-time) and he replies that his last meal was lunch yesterday. The receptionist explains that he should not eat anything now in case he has to be given an anaesthetic for any reason, but that there is nothing to be alarmed about.

The nurse arrives and takes the young man to the doctor who examines the wrist without causing pain. As he thinks, the doctor explains what he believes might have happened in non-technical language. The likelihood is that the wrist is broken, but to be sure and to enable the bone to be set most effectively it will be necessary to take X-rays.

The X-ray confirms that the bone is broken and, after checking that the man has not eaten in the last 24 hours, and after carefully explaining exactly what will happen to him and to his arm, and how he can expect to feel when he comes round, and after gaining the young man's permission, the doctor authorizes the administration of a general anaesthetic. The bone is set.

When he regains consciousness a nurse sits with the young man until he feels well enough to travel home. She explains about the visits he will have to make to the hospital in the future, about how quickly the pain will subside, and about how soon he could be expecting to play football again (not that this is a major anxiety after his last effort). He is given paracetamol for the pain. He is asked whether he drinks, or if he smokes cannabis. The young man says that he is fond of a drink and the nurse tells him that in this case a drink will probably do as well as the paracetamol, but that he should not take both together, which would be dangerous.

What do these two scenarios indicate?

These scenarios go some way towards substantiating the claim that 'work for health is a moral endeavour'.

These scenarios indicate that even in apparently mundane health work interventions—in everyday work for health—the ways in which a person is treated, the degree to which health is created, is inevitably bound up with the degree of morality created. Each of the health workers involved in the scenarios was responsible for intervening directly in another person's life. And although setting bones is an everyday procedure for some health workers it would be a time of crisis in the life of the young man, who would at least be apprehensive about his treatment.

Now all the health workers in the two scenarios had a degree of choice about how they intervened in the situation. They would be bound by contracts of employment, and might wish to conform to professional codes of practice, but even within these boundaries (which as autonomous individuals they could choose to accept or not) a range of personal choice is possible. Dependent upon their choice the physical, emotional, and intellectual consequences might be different for the young man, as is demonstrated by the scenarios.

These observations will be familiar to most people who are interested in everyday activity and who are concerned about their responsibilities to other people. How each of us should behave towards his fellow beings is a central question in ethics. It becomes of even greater importance in the context of health work, which already has the clear rationale of caring for people and helping those who are in trouble in various physical and mental ways.

Hence this conclusion follows. By its very nature health work always involves interventions in the lives of other people. These interventions are made either directly—by a caring touch, by the surgeon's knife, in the consultation, by face to face education—or indirectly—by the hospital administrator deciding which ward to close, by the government ministers agreeing a budget for the health service, by the manager implementing a new policy on nutrition, or by the supervisor deciding upon the best working conditions for staff. But whether these interventions are made directly or indirectly, at some point they have real implications—often major implications—for the lives of other people.

The Key Question

Given this, the *key question*—the question which combines work for health with morality, and which should be the permanent starting point for all health workers—is *'How can I intervene to the highest moral degree?' The key issue is, in each case and in general, what is the highest moral intervention possible?*

If the inquiry is abandoned at this point this key question is so general that it is actually uninformative. One problem is that since different people have different values opinions vary about what is more or less moral, or about what is and what is not moral. Different people can have different ideas, perhaps wildly different ideas, about how to intervene to the highest moral degree.

In order to indicate as clearly as possible what is meant by casting this as the key question a great deal more needs to be said about the nature of ethics, and the nature of different ideas about ethics, than can be given in these introductory chapters. Some people might take 'being ethical' to mean always conforming to a particular view about what is right and what is wrong. If two people hold conflicting opinions about the right and the wrong in particular circumstances then it follows that the interventions they choose to make will also be conflicting and contradictory. Such a situation is common in medicine.

For example, in the case of abortion some doctors take the view that it is simply morally right to abort a foetus if this is the choice of the pregnant woman, while other doctors take the view that it is simply morally wrong to destroy a collection of cells that has the potential to become a human being and a person. In cases such as this it seems futile to advise health workers to deliberate about how to intervene to the most moral degree. The idea of morality seems to be relative, contestable, and irreconcilable, and the idea of intervening morally open to almost any interpretation.

In fact this is not necessarily so. The argument of this book shows that, while the fact that people have different values and that this will lead them to make different choices in their interventions with others is unquestionable, it is possible—taking the view that the essence of morality is the act of deliberating with integrity—to be clear that some interventions in the name of health must be seen as being of a higher moral calibre than others.

As an initial illustration of this point consider the two scenarios above. In both cases work aimed at producing health in the young man produced some degree of morality. The key to understanding which of the scenarios produced the highest degree of morality in its various interventions is to consider the extent to which the various aspects of the young man, as a person rather than merely as a human body with a broken wrist, were repaired, enhanced, or developed.

Even in the rather mundane setting of a casualty department there were a number of opportunities for very different forms of intervention, interventions which could affect the young man physically. intellectually, and emotionally. In both scenarios the wrist was set. But in the first the wrist was set with great and unnecessary pain, and for a significant period the young man suffered uncertainty and anxiety: partly as a result of the receptionist's failure to inform him not to eat the boiled sweets and partly because he was not listened to by other staff, and because nothing was explained to him. In the second scenario attention was paid to the young man's physical comfort, and time was also spent to enable him to understand his circumstances and the future development of his wrist. He was also helped to feel emotionally calm and generally safe.

In the first scenario the young man was enabled in a physical sense. This was both an intention and a consequence. But there was no attempt to enable him to understand, or to be reassured, and there was no intention—no need seen—to respect his opinions, feelings, or wishes. The idea seems to have been that these were either irrelevant or wrong, or both. In the second scenario the wrist was set, and so in this scenario too the man was enabled physically. But in this case he was also educated, his immediate emotional needs were detected and addressed, and he was treated with respect. He was asked his choice after options were explained to him.

It is possible to conclude provisionally, without the argument of the remainder of this book, that the interventions which took place in the second scenario were of a higher moral standard than those which took place in the first (reference to the *Ethical Grid* will indicate how such a position might be justified).

Other Important Questions and Topics

The identification of the central question for health work is only part of the initial task. The central question for health workers—'*How can I intervene to the highest moral degree?*'—is not a catch-all question. It is not always the most appropriate question to ask, but it is a highly useful overall guide to the other sorts of questions that need to be posed and borne in mind. It is important to highlight a number of significant areas which have to be considered by thoughtful health workers.

Central topics

The priority for a serious inquiry is to ensure that the questions asked are the most central possible. By posing the right questions and opening up the central topic areas it is possible to grasp the soul of the puzzle. These questions and topic areas are discussed again at the conclusion of this book.

The central areas to be borne in mind during the remainder of this book are the following.

1. How can we work to create more health when we do not:

(*a*) *know for certain what health is*?

(b) *agree between ourselves what health is*?

These issues need to be resolved. Significant progress has been made (Seedhouse 1986) through the use of philosophical analysis of both ideas and practice. The present account is in many ways a natural development of this earlier work. By focusing explicitly on the moral content of work for health this book makes real agreement about the nature of health, and the limits to work for health, more likely.

2. How can we be ethical when we do not:

(a) *know for certain what it is to be ethical*?

(b) *agree between ourselves what it is to be ethical*?

These questions are of vital importance for this analysis. Without proper clarification of the nature of ethics, without some clear idea about the different possible views about ethics, it is simply not possible to reach any decision about the morality of interventions. And practically, without understanding of the limits of what is moral and what is not moral, there need be no end to the actions that people might 'justify' as moral. There is a vast area of possible activity and intervention that is not specifically covered by legislation. Consequently there is a need for guidelines about the nature of morality. But these guidelines should not be finally binding and always prescriptive. They should be indicators of the limit to the moral realm.

3. The nature of interventions

(a) *What is an intervention? What types of intervention are there*?

It is possible to distinguish a variety of types of intervention. For example, there are clear differences of kind and moral implication between:

  (i) An intervention that is requested and agreed. For example, the intervention that takes place when a person consults his general practitioner voluntarily.
 (ii) An intervention that is not requested but which the client desires, or finds desirable. For example, the intervention that takes place when a health visitor or district nurse calls unannounced and finds an old lady alone without heating, and too proud to ask for help.
(iii) An intervention that is not requested and not desired. For example, the sort of intervention that might take place when a health professional visits the house of a smoker to explain why he should stop. Or an intervention by a consultant to do controlled tests on drugs in groups of patients without their knowledge.
 (iv) An intervention that is enforced by law. For example, interventions to quarantine those people with notifiable diseases, compulsory sterilization of teenage girls defined as being mentally sub-normal, or interventions to detain persons under Sections of the Mental Health Act, 1983.
  (v) Not intervening through neglect. For example, a social worker failing to notice signs of child abuse is sometimes an omission that has major consequences.

(vi) Radical non-intervention. For example, sometimes in social work decisions are taken not to intervene where interventions would normally be made. For instance, it may be judged that the risk of intervening in families on some 'volatile' housing estates is too great.

(b) *In what ways can interventions be justified?*

The intention of the person who is to intervene, and the predicted and actual consequences of the intervention have to be considered in order to understand the morality of the intervention. For example, it might be argued that the degree of morality of the consultant testing drugs on patients without their knowledge will be different dependent on his motive and on the potential or actual benefits and dangers to other people.

(c) *What is the difference (if any) between an intervention that raises ethical issues and an intervention that does not?*

It might be thought that a clear distinction could be made between interventions that raise a moral dimension and those that are morally neutral, In fact, as this book shows, it is doubtful whether such a basic distinction can ever be sustained.

4. How can a clear limit to health interventions be set out? How can this limit be informative and useful without imposing rigid rules and codes on health workers? The Ethical Grid is one attempt at answering this question.

5. What is a person? What is a full person? This is a central topic because the idea of 'persons' helps make it clear why we should regard people as important. It helps clarify why we bother to work for health at all, and why the notion of morality is central to civilization. It is possible to distinguish between a person in a basic sense, and full persons. Work for health, moral work, is work to ensure that there are more full persons in the world.

The Stage is Set

The problem has been outlined. The problem is that health workers need to find some way of ensuring that health care in the future is of the best possible kind. A path towards an answer has been sketched out. The answer involves the knowledge that an understanding of ethics can provide the key. Initial distinctions have been made within the field of ethics, and a central question has been identified. Thus the stage is set for the inquiry proper to begin, for case studies to be presented, and for a means of coping with these case studies (the Ethical Grid) to be offered.

Chapter Four
Problems of Practice

Introduction

The crisis—be it real or a graphic device—is not merely about what is, about what things can be done and what things can be done better. It is about what *ought* to be. What ought to be is a driving issue in moral philosophy. Consequently both a theoretical and a practical solution to the question of what ought to be requires systematic critical analysis. That such an analysis is necessary is shown by these case studies, which, although most appear to be mundane, pose huge moral and practical problems.

All these examples of practice raise choices. Health workers manage already to deal with practical choices. It would be unjust and arrogant to argue that a contribution from philosophy is essential, that without clarification nothing can ever be resolved. Rather the aim is to improve the skills of health workers in this aspect of their work, by providing knowledge and understanding of ethical reasoning and how to apply it.

Given that a major theme of this book is that at present the focus of health work is limited by an overemphasis on the elimination and prevention of disease and illness, and that the medical definition of health is not rich enough, it might appear strange that all the case studies outlined in this chapter are linked to issues of disease and illness, even though they are exactly the sort of problems that health workers must confront at present.

All interventions are moral or immoral to some degree. There are four reasons for focusing on the type of case study described in this chapter, rather than on case studies that raise issues about education, or about distribution of warm and safe housing, or about the creation of secure and fulfilling employment. These reasons are:

1. The case studies have a clear relevance and interest for present health workers.
2. Medical work against disease and illness is a genuine part of work for health and will remain so.
3. The paradigm change is by no means complete. These case studies help to show that within present health work there are elements of both the fading paradigm and the new era.
4. By focusing on the current practice of health workers it might be possible to accelerate the paradigm change by showing that a far richer theory of health needs to be clearly and overtly acknowledged.

The practical problems of intervention which challenge health workers are presented in case studies, none of which has an answer that is 'obviously right'. That is, an answer that anyone and everyone can agree about. Any answer offered in response to a case study will require justification and explanation. Why this solution and not other possibilities? There are always alternative courses of action—often several alternative courses of action—open to the health professionals and other participants in each of the studies.

In this chapter the studies are presented without attempt at analysis of the ethical issues. This is partly to do with the way in which this inquiry is organized and presented, and partly for educational reasons. It will be a useful exercise for any interested reader to write down the course of action that she would take or advise, together with her reasons for it and any criticisms of the alternatives. Alternatively she could simply write down her feelings and intuitions about the case. It will be enlightening to consider later, when the nature of ethics and the reasoning behind various ethical theories has been explained in more detail, whether personal understanding of the principles underlying each option, and understanding of and justification for individual proposals and solutions, has been enlarged. It might even be that opinions change and thought develops as a result of the clarification contained in later chapters. If so this will be an indication of the success of applied philosophy.

The Case Studies

Every case study raises a range of issues. Not all of these issues will be immediately apparent. After each study tasks are suggested for those who wish to explore the moral issues for themselves.

1. Teaching or caring: Michael and Caroline

Michael is a health visitor. He is devoted to his profession because he feels that it allows him to do professionally what he would wish to do voluntarily. He believes passionately that the primary reason for any person's existence is to help other people. Michael lives to care. He is a sensitive man who empathizes naturally with nearly everyone he meets. He has the gift of seeing life as other people see it. He can shift easily into the perspectives of the people he cares for. Michael often says that the secret of good health visiting is 'to be able to step temporarily into the other person's shoes'. Some of his many friends worry that sometimes Michael's temporary becomes a little too permanent.

The seeds of the problem were sown during Michael's time as a health visitor student. An incident that happened at the end of his training upset Michael profoundly, so much so that he was not able to articulate fully all the aspects which distressed him. As part of his fieldwork experience Michael was assigned an elderly lady to visit once a month between October and June. Caroline was 79, a widow, rather frail but still able to cook and clean. She had a home help twice a week. She had no disease, and the only medication she needed was a tumbler of neat whisky every evening. Caroline could reflect on a rich life. She had married twice, once to a journalist. Her other husband had been a businessman. She had been able to travel widely with both, meeting an enormous variety of people on the way, and had written about her experiences in two books. Her problem now was loneliness. Her last husband had died three years earlier, and she still missed him desperately.

Michael did not see his health visiting role from a medical perspective. His brief from his supervisor was to observe and support Caroline. He did not consider himself primarily as a nurse making sure that Caroline did not suffer physical illness and injury, even though he recognized this to be an important role for a health visitor in many contexts. Rather Michael felt that his role was to befriend the widow, to help her see the past with fondness instead of regret and hopeless longing, to help her focus on the talents and possibilities that still remained open to her, and to encourage her to share herself with other people. Over the months Michael and Caroline became friends, despite the 45 year gap in their ages. Caroline had begun, although the process had been slow, to think about what she could do now rather than what she had done in the past. As for Michael, he was pleased with what he was achieving with Caroline, and he too had developed. Caroline had built up a hard edge, a cynicism, during her dealings with people in journalism and business. Her stories, her accounts of her decisions and of the politics of life, saddened the committed altruist, but he recognized a certain truth in what she was saying, a necessity about what she had done. Michael was benefiting too.

The problem was that, for reasons his superior refused to outline, Michael was assigned a different case load when he qualified, even though he was still operating the same 'patch' as before. Michael explained that he believed that he was doing useful work with Caroline, and what was more he was enjoying it, and thought it right to continue. All his supervisor would say was that the old lady's circumstances did not merit the services of a busy health visitor. She was in truth useful only as part of the 'learning experience'. Michael said that in that case he would continue to visit Caroline in a private capacity, but his supervisor replied curtly that this would not be advisable. It would be an 'unprofessional' action.

Exercise

- List the key issues as they occur.
- State approval or disapproval of the interventions made in this study.
- Suggest ways in which any interventions made in this study could achieve a higher degree of morality.
- Justify any opinions and suggestions.

---

2. Telling the truth?

Two health education officers, Barbara and Kim, have been instructed to launch a campaign to improve local people's diets. They work in a small department under a district health education officer. The department is based in an inner-city area in the north west of England, so the two officers are familiar with the high levels of unemployment, avoidable disease, and general deprivation. Both Barbara and Kim are Social Science graduates and well-equipped to research their subject area.

The District Medical Officer, who is the direct superior to the District Health Education Officer and responsible for policy decisions, has instructed that the campaign must be based solely on the guidelines presented in a recently published booklet. Barbara and Kim consider what to do. Kim knows immediately that she must, as a responsible and professional health education officer, carry out her brief to the letter. But Barbara has a number of worries.

Barbara is concerned about the following aspects. First, she soon discovered that the booklet received 50 per cent of its funding from the Health Education Authority, and the other half from the butter industry.

Secondly, Barbara's conclusion is that although the booklet is sumptuously produced—colourful, graphic, and glossy—it is very hard to read. It is not clear what the practical advice actually is. Barbara wonders whether it is possible that the information has been presented in this way deliberately in order to confuse, so that people stick with their present habits. She cannot be sure of the intentions of the writers and artists, but she is concerned about the results that the booklet will have. Thirdly, from her research she has learnt that some of the information (in this case especially about fats) is significantly incomplete, to the extent that a biased picture appears to have been presented. Fourthly, Barbara is not at all sure that the information and the advice—the 'facts'—given in the booklet are necessarily the truth. Much of it seems to be opinion rather than certainty, and to propagate opinion in the guise of fact seems to Barbara to be simple propaganda. And she does not want to be involved in a propaganda exercise.

Barbara has spent time researching the history of nutrition research and advice and realizes that much depends upon the fashions of the time, the social trends of a particular era, the types of foods that are available, and the amount of money that people have to spend on food. Also she has read alternative theories to those presented in the booklet, and she knows that informed commentators dispute several of the claims made in the booklet.

A further point noticed by Barbara is that when the nature of the geographic area in which she and Kim must campaign is taken into account, it becomes questionable whether the campaign will be effective. It might be a simple waste of time and money. The people living in nearby tower blocks, in damp, noisy, and crowded conditions, unable to find work, and under considerable pressure from life's iniquitous burdens are unlikely to change the comforting habits of a lifetime because of glossy advice delivered by a pair of reasonably well-off, middle-class health education officers.

Barbara explains her worries and findings to Kim, who listens and understands what she is being told, but none the less insists on doing her duty as a health education officer working for the health service. She can do no other than defer to the opinion of a qualified medic.

Exercise
- List the key issues as they occur.
- Which of the health education officers is attempting to intervene with the highest degree of morality?
- What should Barbara do? How can she intervene in practice with the highest degree of morality?
- Justify any opinions and suggestions.

---

3. To immunize or not?

Diane is a health visitor employed by a health authority. The authority has a policy on immunization and vaccination. It is chaired by an ambitious man who likes to win. He is determined that his district will return the best vaccination figures in the country. Essentially he sees the task as a sales campaign and each employee as an agent for the policy, as a sales representative. The policy is also advocated strongly by the Specialist in Community Medicine (Child Health), and pressure is brought to bear on all the local general practitioners to ensure that they are as effective as possible in the campaign. The health visitors are seen as the main sales representatives and educators. It is possible for them to exert very strong pressure on clients—for instance, on mothers whose children are due for immunization. Such phrases as 'go on, its the right thing to do', 'you really must agree, all the other mums have', and 'its only fair on the child, you know' can be very powerful when said to women who are uncertain what to do and who want the best for their children.

The target is a straightforward 100 per cent uptake for all those who show no contra-indications. The main thrust of this particular campaign is set against whooping cough. Diane has been instructed to convince every parent or guardian of the children she visits that the vaccination is definitely in the interest of each child. But Diane has doubts. She has researched the subject and, against the current tide of opinion, has arrived at the view that the risks of immunization outweigh the benefits (Office of Health Economics 1974), and that this is what the campaign ought to be saying, while at the same time offering the service to those who wish it. Diane knows that she would not choose to have her child vaccinated, and so she cannot honestly advocate vaccination.

Diane decides first that she is not prepared to run the risk of directly inflicting injury upon another human being. She would prefer instead to make sure that each child is fit, well housed, and well nourished, and so better able to cope with whooping cough if it strikes. Secondly, Diane is opposed to a high pressure sales campaign because she is not prepared to frighten another human being unnecessarily, or to inflict stress and guilt upon a human being who refuses to cooperate.

Diane's dilemma is that as a professional working for the State she has a duty to follow the instructions she has been given. If she fails to do this she must accept the consequence of probable dismissal, and even legal action if a parent can show that Diane gave false or misleading information. Yet as a person in her own right, with opinions which she feels that she can justify, Diane believes that she should pursue an alternative policy. She believes that to implement the campaign is deceitful and possibly dangerous, and that there will be less overall benefit from it than there would be from her suggested option.

She feels that the true hub of this issue is actually not to do with whether it is better to immunize. The evidence for and against is uncertain, and there is a risk associated with vaccination that no one can honestly deny. Given this uncertainty Diane sees that what is at stake is how people treat their fellow men. She is, she believes, being asked to lie, to coerce, and to treat adults as if they are children who can cope only with simplicities and one side of the story. She does not wish to be party to a mass insult against the local people, even if it is genuinely and honestly intended to be for the good of the population as a whole. What is 'good' is arguable, and Diane thinks in this case there are a number of possible candidates for the title 'supreme good'. Among these is the notion of respect for fellow men, and regarding other people as intellectually valuable and autonomous, or potentially autonomous. She would cast this 'good', on this occasion, above the 'good' of preventing physical harm.

An associated point that Diane takes into account is that middle-class children are vaccinated to raise herd immunity, although those children are not in personal need of the immunization. This is never explained to their parents for fear that they might refuse, even though it would be far more respectful and honest to explain that the immunization could be done for the sake of others.

Exercise

In this case study it is possible to focus attention only on Diane, which is why her beliefs have been explained in such detail. What should Diane do to achieve the highest moral intervention in this case? Before listing options and justifying them it is important to note that Diane appears to have some straightforward options, and faces a difficult decision.

Should Diane:

- Obey the rules as behoves a professional? If it is believed that it is right for these rules to be obeyed against her judgement, what sorts of rules should be disobeyed? For instance, should professionals obey any rules that are part of their job description? Should they lie? Steal? Coerce? Kill?
- Resign or be sacked? In either case she could be sure that someone else would come along and follow the rules in her stead.
- Manipulate the system so that she achieved the end that she believed to be the most moral, whilst remaining in the job?

---

4. Two case studies concerning AIDS

(a) **Social control and individual rights—what price do you pay?**   This situation, which is at present only hypothetical, might soon become reality. The following extract appeared in the *Observer* newspaper in Britain on 31 August 1986 under the story heading 'Wild Man of the Right leads drive for A.I.D.S. apartheid':

> Doctors, public health officials, and political leaders in California last week denounced as 'hateful and absurd' a proposal which could lead to mandatory blood tests for anyone suspected of carrying the A.I.D.S. virus.
>
> Under the measure, known as Proposition 64, thousands of A.I.D.S. sufferers could be isolated, quarantined, barred from schools, restaurants and other public places, and possibly tatooed for identification.
>
> 'It raises the spectre of concentration camps for A.I.D.S. patients,' said Bruce Decker, head of a state advisory committee on the disease, 'which is where the sponsors of this wretched proposal really want them put.'

Proposition 64 was defeated 2:1 in a ballot on 4 November 1986. However, it is unlikely that this will be the last proposal of its sort placed before legislative bodies. The case for such proposals is straightforward. First, it seems unquestionable that the most effective way of eliminating the AIDS virus is to isolate or destroy every carrier and sufferer in order that no further transmissions are possible. The virus would then die with its hosts. Secondly, it is a fundamental principle of most State constitutions that innocent people are entitled to protection from threats to life.

The first premise is probably true. But this does not mean that there are not other means available of controlling or halting the AIDS epidemic that are effective. The second premise could be read as implying that those people who carry the virus are somehow guilty of having committed a moral crime or a crime in law. Or if it does not it argues that a small group of innocent people should be sacrificed in order to protect the majority of innocent people who have the good fortune not to have the AIDS disease. Propositions such as Proposition 64 propose that the rights of a minority of individuals should be simply abrogated for the good of the majority.

This type of proposition is an example of a crude form of consequentialism where, so long as the overall balance for mankind is an increase of good consequences over evil consequences, then the action leading to those consequences can be morally justified. But there is a huge price to be paid for this. The notion of justice, where it is considered to be a moral wrong if people who are fundamentally equal in their beings are treated, for any reason, as if they are basically unequal, has to be forgotten.

- In this case the 'health intervention' will be made initially at the level of government or local government. But the choice made by a legislative body between this extreme solution and the range of alternatives must have clear and direct implications for individuals and communities. The type of intervention laid out in Proposition 64 could set a precedent for the ways in which other communicable diseases are dealt with. Health professionals would be at the sharp end of the interventions and need to form opinions about where lines are to be drawn. If it is acceptable to quarantine the victims of AIDS for the good of the majority then it should also be acceptable to quarantine those people with venereal disease, those with influenza, and those with measles. What is acceptable?

Exercise

- List other key issues as they occur.
- State approval or disapproval of Proposition 64.
- Consider alternative interventions which might achieve a higher degree of morality.
- Justify any opinions and suggestions.

(b) The general practitioner and the government campaign   Dr George is a general practitioner working in a typical suburb of Birmingham in England. Along with all other English GPs he has been sent the information on AIDS prepared by the government and the Health Education Council (later Health Education Authority). He has read this information and has been alarmed by it. He understands that:

> Any man or woman can get the Aids virus depending on their behaviour.
>   It is not just a homosexual disease.
>   There is no cure. And it kills.
>   By the time you read this, probably 300 people will have died in this country. It is believed that a further 30 000 carry the virus. This number is rising and will continue to rise unless we all take precautions. 'Aids: Don't die of ignorance' Government Information leaflet, January 1987.

Dr George understands that the AIDS virus can be transmitted through the blood of an infected person entering another person's body via an open wound, and through semen during sexual intercourse. He knows that male homosexuals and drug users who share needles are groups at high risk of becoming infected with the AIDS virus.

Occasionally the question of AIDS is raised by patients. Most of these are concerned that their past sexual activities might mean that they are carriers of the virus. Paul, a heterosexual man of 25, consulted Dr George to ask for a human immunodeficiency test (a test to detect the presence of antibodies to a virus which causes the acquired immune deficiency syndrome). He told him that during his time at university he had 'made love' to several women and that he was worried that he might have AIDS because he knew that they too had been 'sleeping around'. Dr George, who is happily married, a Methodist, and in his early fifties, arranged the test. But he also decided to lecture Paul, quite severely and for ten minutes, about his sexual activities. Dr George repeatedly said that what Paul chose to do was entirely Paul's own business, but that to continue with this sort of behaviour now that the extent of the AIDS threat was known was highly dangerous. Paul should stick to one partner. Dr George wanted to know why Paul didn't find a nice girl and settle down now that he was 25.

Paul began to suffer great anxiety after this consultation. He worked himself up into such an emotional state that he became quite convinced that he had AIDS. Before he took the test he became so stressed that he was unable to do his job properly. He returned to the practice after three days for a further consultation. This time he was seen by Dr Phillips. Paul explained his difficulties to Dr Phillips, an unmarried woman in her early thirties. She took a very different approach from Dr George.

Dr Phillips had also seen the government information about AIDS, but through diligent reading of the medical journals had reached different conclusions. She did not feel that she could justify merely transmitting to patients the information presented by the government. She felt that as a professional she had a fundamental responsibility to establish, as far as possible, the veracity of the government information. Dr Phillips discovered that although the AIDS virus has been *found* in both cervical and vaginal secretions it is not certain that the virus can be effectively *transmitted* through this route. She also discovered that up to the end of 1986 there were only ten cases of men having apparently picked up the virus through heterosexual contact, and that only one of the cases picked up the infection in Britain.

Dr Phillips explained her findings to Paul, who was at first incredulous and then highly relieved. Dr Phillips documented her sources for Paul and said that he could check for himself in the local university library. Dr Phillips also offered to cancel the test for the human immunodeficiency virus. Paul said that he would let her know his decision as soon as he had considered the further reading she had suggested.

Exercise

- List the key issues as they occur.
- State approval or disapproval of the interventions made in this study.
- Suggest ways in which any interventions made in this study could achieve a higher degree of morality.
- Justify any opinions and suggestions.

5. Sponsorship and hidden motives

Professor Ronson is head of a Department of Community Medicine. He wants his department to be involved in as many research projects which will benefit the community as possible. Professor Ronson also wishes to employ as many research staff as possible since he appreciates that it is becoming increasingly difficult for researchers to find posts at British universities and polytechnics. Professor Ronson has an idea for a research project to discover the reasons why there is a relatively low use of the medical and health facilities, including a health centre and a well-women's centre, in one part of the city. The uptake rate was expected to be fairly low because the area in question is the poorest in the district, with the highest levels of unemployment and single-parent families. However, the precise reasons for the lack of use of the facilities are not known. Considering that the local population suffers a disproportionately high level of disease and illness it seems to be unquestionably important to understand more about why the people act as they do.

The controversy begins at this point. Professor Ronson has exhausted his research budget so he makes it known to potential sponsors and research bodies that he wishes to embark on a two-year project, employing at least one research associate. Unfortunately for the professor, none of the usual sources of funds wishes to or is able to help. However, out of the blue there comes an offer of sponsorship from a famous tobacco company. The company tells Professor Ronson that it intends to fund worthwhile health research throughout the country and is pleased to say that this is one of its first offers.

The nature of this dilemma is very clear: should Professor Ronson accept the sponsorship from a company which trades in a commodity which creates disease and illness?

Exercise

- List the key issues as they occur.
- State approval or disapproval of the interventions made in this study.
- Suggest ways in which any interventions made in this study could achieve a higher degree of morality.
- Justify any opinions and suggestions.

---

6. Tragic choices

Unlike the other case studies described so far where alternative courses of action are possible, this study is at the 'sharp end' of moral philosophy—at the tip of the iceberg. It poses the type of dilemma most commonly felt to typify the raw material on which moral philosophers work. The dilemma is set up in such a way that there are two (or sometimes more) possible choices to make. Both choices could be justified. But whichever option is chosen there will always be a price to pay that could have been prevented if the other option had been chosen. The French philosopher Jean-Paul Sartre gave the following example of a tragic choice: in the Second World War a young man has to make a choice between leaving home to fight with the French Resistance movement striving to free France from German occupation, or staying at home to protect and look after his frail mother who would have to live alone if he were to leave. What is the young man to do?

The reason that there are not more case studies of the 'tragic choice' kind included in this book is that such cases are exceptional, and not the everyday experience of health workers. A central argument of this analysis is that every intervention in the life of another person will be moral or immoral to some degree. There are no neutral interventions. Occasionally health workers will be faced with 'tragic choices' and so it is useful to have some experience in dealing with these.

The nurse practitioner's dilemma   This study concerns a nurse practitioner. Nurse practitioners are nurses who work from health centres, and whom patients can consult as an alternative to seeing the doctor. They can recommend some treatments and can refer the patient on to the doctor if necessary. Many in nursing see the advent of nurse practitioners as an important step in increasing the status of the nursing profession.

Sandra is a pioneering nurse practitioner who has quickly built up a list of patients who find it easier to deal with her than with the doctors. The doctors who also work in the practice do not resent this since they recognize the benefit of Sandra's presence both to themselves and to the patients.

Sandra is about to attend a vital national meeting in which a proposal to extend the nurse practitioner programme to all parts of the country is either to be agreed or rejected. As an articulate pioneer her attendance is crucial. It will mean the difference between nurse practitioners becoming a recognized part of the NHS or remaining as exceptions for the foreseeable future, on the periphery of health care.

As Sandra is about to leave for the meeting the receptionist rushes to tell her that one of her patients is on the phone threatening to commit suicide and insists on seeing her. Sandra knows that the patient is highly strung and sensitive, and she knows that very probably she is the only one who will be able to help. Sandra could be directly responsible for saving the distraught woman's life.

The dilemma is this: should Sandra stay to help the person who is threatening to end her life, or should she go to the meeting to ensure that more nurse practitioners become available to help many more people, and possibly save many more lives?

Exercise

- List the key issues as they occur.
- State approval or disapproval of the options for intervening that are open to Sandra.
- Suggest which of the options for intervening would achieve the higher degree of morality.
- Justify any opinions and suggestions.

---

7. Is coercion acceptable?

What is coercion?   Coercion can be thought of as constraining or compelling a person into thinking or doing something she would not otherwise have done. Coercion involves the control either entirely or in part of an otherwise autonomous being.

The question is this: Is it ever right to coerce a person, either for what is perceived to be that person's own good, or for the good of society or mankind as a whole? This single question inevitably raises a number of others. For example, Is coercion *always* undesirable? Can coercion be justified and if so on what ground? What factors should be taken into consideration before the imposition of, for instance, a medically defined 'good' on another person? Is there an implication that the one who intends to coerce possesses esoteric or superior knowledge which it is impossible or not desirable to transmit to the person who is to be coerced? If so, does this imply that the coerced does not have, or cannot be permitted to have, the ability to choose, and that the ability of the coercer is superior in this respect?

The forthright district nurse   Anne is a district nurse with strong views against smoking. These views have become firmly dogmatic over the last six months because Anne has had to visit two families whose lives have been thrown into temporary chaos as a result of one member of each (in one case the mother and in the other the father) dying from lung cancer. Both the deceased parents had smoked over 30 cigarettes per day consistently for many years.

In Anne's opinion there is simply no question that both deaths were directly attributable to the smoking habits. Both people would still be alive, in all probability for 20 or so more years, if they had not smoked. Anne has developed a strategy to deal with the smoking problem if it exists in other families that she has to visit in future.

Anne regards smoking as a simple evil which ought to be totally stamped out. She does not believe that smoking has any benefits at all, and she does not make any distinction between types of smoker on any ground. More developed views than Anne's are possible. For example, one might distinguish between those whose habit harms no one else and those who are smoking in homes shared by young families; and it is also possible to distinguish between those who wish to give up and those smokers who believe that smoking is helpful to them in some way. Perhaps they are very tense and nervous and smoking helps them to relax, and they consider that the side-effects of smoking are a price worth paying for this relaxation. But Anne's aim is to stop the habit, whatever the reasons people have for smoking.

These are the stages through which her strategy is designed to progress:

First, she always makes it clear that on no account is smoking permitted during her visit to the home.

Secondly, Anne states emphatically that there is absolutely no doubt that smoking causes cancer.

Thirdly, Anne offers, and always leaves anyway, anti-smoking pamphlets and information about why it is foolish to smoke.

Fourthly, Anne deliberately changes her attitude from friendliness to hostility when she knows that one of her clients is continuing to smoke despite her advice.

Finally, if her patient continues to refuse to cooperate then Anne's strategy is the severest she can apply. For a time Anne continues to provide the minimum treatment necessary for the condition, but she makes it clear that she could do more. If even this fails to produce the desired result Ann refuses treatment to whichever member of the family is in need of it until the smoker, even it it is not the patient him or herself, gives up.

Exercise

(Note: it is important to consider the law in this case.)

- List the key issues as they occur.
- State approval or disapproval of Anne's strategy for intervention.
- Suggest ways of increasing the degree of morality of this anti-smoking intervention (if there are any).
- Justify any opinions and suggestions.

---

8. Death and the truth

Jane is an experienced nurse who works on a mixed ward which caters mainly for cancer sufferers at various stages of their treatments. Jane is a Catholic and very single-minded about telling the truth. She believes that everybody has a basic right to information about themselves and the circumstances in which they find themselves. And when the relevant information is that they will soon be dead Jane believes that she has a simple duty to tell her patients because they will then have the opportunity to prepare themselves, their relatives, and their friends, and they will be able to make their peace with God. Jane believes that her duty extends to telling people this information even though the patient is avoiding the issue, and even if the medical judgement is that the knowledge would cause 'psychological damage'.

Is Jane right in her policy? Is giving this information the most ethical intervention possible in this situation?

Exercise

- List the key issues as they occur.
- State approval or disapproval of Jane's policy.
- Suggest alternative policies for intervention in this context which would create a higher degree of morality.
- Justify any opinions and suggestions.

---

9. Is all drug education health education?

Kathy is a thoughtful and conscientious health education officer. Her District Health Education Officer has decided that Kathy will be responsible for the local campaign against 'drug misuse'. Kathy believes that some of this material is misleading in various ways. Some is clearly designed to shock. For example, death, or physical disability, or a zombie-like existence, is predicted starkly by the use of posters as an inevitable consequence of 'drug misuse'. Further, as it appears to Kathy, some of the material sets out to create such myths as: the smoking of cannabis will lead inevitably to the smoking or injecting of heroin; experimenting with heroin means instant dependency for the user; illegal drugs are the only truly dangerous drugs; all illegal drugs are equally liable to create dependency; the use of drugs means that the user will eventually be unable to hold down work, or unable to have a social life with people who do not use drugs. And yet further, the information Kathy has been asked to distribute pays insufficient attention, in Kathy's opinion, to the fact that a major cause of dependency arises from addiction to prescribed drugs such as tranquillizers (which can create a dependency from which it is unpleasant and difficult to withdraw if they are taken regularly over months). ('Britain's Innocent Addicts', *The Observer*, Sunday 28 February 1988).

Kathy is a person who hates the thought that a person's major interest in life is finding ways in which to escape it. She is strongly in favour of preventing dependency on drugs and of offering alternative means for people to find life worthwhile, but she is strongly opposed to deception and gross exaggeration of information presented as 'the truth', whatever the motivation of the person who seeks to deceive. Kathy is also very disturbed that, directly and explicitly, she has become an agent for the government. This need not necessarily be a bad thing but, in terms of lack of autonomy and control over what she does, Kathy believes that there is real cause for concern. Kathy outlined her fears to the District Health Education Officer who referred her to the District Medical Officer, who told her kindly that she must do as she is told by her superior. This means in practice that Kathy is obliged by her employer to ensure that the posters are placed in public libraries and other public places; and that Kathy must face a tricky decision over the content of her lectures about drugs to groups of teenagers. She is supposed to follow the official line but she knows (she is only 24) that this strategy will be ineffective and even counter-productive with such groups, many of whom will have tried, and almost certainly will know people who have tried, illegal drugs and not experienced in reality the tales of horror that she has been told to frighten them with. And she must also face a related problem—which boils down to a question of personal integrity—when she has to present a talk to a group of parents, many of whom will expect to have the government hyperbole confirmed.

Exercise

- List the key issues as they occur to you.
- Suggest a form of intervention which will create the highest degree of morality.
- Justify any opinions and suggestions.

---

10. It's for your own good

This case study is about the addition of fluoride to the national water supply. It could equally well concern the implementation of any policy done 'in the interests of the people' without consultation of 'the people'.

The background is straightforward. In order to decrease levels of tooth decay, in some areas of the country fluoride is introduced directly into the public water supply, so that if a person drinks water he will also contact a chemical added by other people who intend that his teeth should be in as good a condition as possible.

Discussion   There are two immediate levels of debate to address. The first concerns the empirical evidence about fluoride. In what ways, if any, is the addition of fluoride to the water supply, good for teeth? Some researchers argue that the effects are neutral or even harmful to people, although most of the research evidence at the moment indicates that the addition of fluoride is of benefit.

The second level of debate concerns opinion about 'the ethics' of this sort of intervention. This level can never be legitimately discussed independently of the first. A central conflict is frequently perceived to exist between the demand that people ought to have full control over their own lives, making all important decisions for themselves, and the fact that, in a complex modern society, many generally beneficial policies can be implemented only at a collective, national level. And this is a level of intervention where it is not possible to consult with all the individuals who will be affected by it.

The general issue raised by the fluoridation debate is this: if fluoridation of the water supply is acceptable, and is explicitly acceptable as an intervention that is 'good' for a population when the 'good' has been defined by the few who have both knowledge and power, then what other 'goods' is it acceptable to impose on populations? Where is the line to be drawn? (This issue is discussed in Seedhouse 1986, pp. 64–8).

Are the following measures justifiable in terms of the production of a 'good' for the population taken as a whole: obligatory sterilization for certain minorities, for instance, the mentally sub-normal, or promiscuous girls; enforced employment on community projects for certain groups, for instance, the long-term unemployed; conscription into the national army; the raising of nutritional standards and norms by prohibiting the sale of 'junk food'; a ban on the sale of tobacco and alcohol; mandatory immunization; the creation of sanitation and hygiene inspectors for domestic homes with powers to enforce whatever recommendations they decide to make; enforced quarantine for all people suffering from infectious diseases; medication and/or incarceration for those people who, whether defined as mentally ill or deviant, have opinions that are considered to be abnormal and likely to threaten the stability of society; specific 'moral education' designed to ensure that traditional family life and values are maintained in the cause of 'the good of all'? Where is the line to be drawn?

Conclusion to Chapter Four

This chapter has presented a range of different case studies focusing on the sorts of situations that are faced by health workers daily, and has ended with a study that has highlighted the association of health with liberty. In this way this chapter serves both as teaching material and as a vital route into the issues and discussion of the rest of this book.

Most of the case studies have not been dramatic ethical dilemmas, of the sort most commonly associated with ethics. Many have been apparently rather mundane, even to the point where it might be difficult at first to see that the studies relate to ethics at all. But each, when analysed and thought through, can be seen to raise moral questions of immense significance. All health workers—nurses, doctors, auxiliaries, chaplins, social workers, non-medical staff, consultants, managers, teachers, administrators, and patients—are involved in daily intervention and interaction that is moral or immoral to some degree. The secret is to recognize this. Once a health worker is aware of the extent to which morality impregnates her work she can take steps to ensure that she directs her activity towards increasing morality in everyday situations.

These 'mundane' case studies ultimately raise issues that the more 'dramatic' case studies (for instance, Case 4a and Case 10, where the tensions between 'the interest of the individual' and 'the interest of the community' are explicit) make more immediately apparent. The issue that is to feature throughout the remainder of this investigation, in a variety of forms, concerns the now clear connection between the ideas of *health* and *liberty*. Such an association of ideas becomes inevitable once the implications of the sorts of health work interventions described in the case studies are made clear. Some means of weighing up which price one should pay, of deliberating over the most moral way to act, of deciding whether one's priority should be the cure of disease or the creation of more personal liberty (if these ideas are in conflict), urgently needs to be found.

Part II

'Hunting the moral'

Chapter Five
The Search for Morality

Introduction

The key question for health workers has been discovered. It is this: How can I intervene to the highest moral degree? In order to give good practical answers to this question during everyday interventions it is necessary for health workers to understand more about the nature of morality. It has already been said that 'being moral' is not simply a matter of 'doing the right thing' where there is just one right course of action and one wrong way. Ethics is complex.

It has also been said that the degree of morality achieved during interventions is linked to the degree of enhancing human potential liberated by the intervention. This is a fairly adequate theoretical guide for health workers, but more needs to be clarified, more needs to be made concrete, if health workers are to be able to apply the theory in practice.

Consequently it is important to attempt to search for morality. If we can have clear examples of what it is to be moral, then it may be possible to extrapolate from these a guide to ethical behaviour. During the course of this chapter this hope will be dashed. But a solid base from which to work morally will be given nevertheless, although its source will be surprising.

The basic difficulty involved with the search for the truly moral arises because people have beliefs and values which conflict, and which cannot be tested for truth or falsity. The statement 'water boils at 100 degrees Celsius at sea level' is testable, it can be proved to be true provided the definitions included in it, and the method of testing, are agreed. It is an empirical matter. But the statement 'it is right to perform euthanasia on a patient who has expressed this wish three years previously' cannot be tested. It might be possible to establish whether or not the patient actually expressed this wish three years ago, but it is not possible to discover empirically whether or not the health worker is *right* to assist with the request.

In this chapter this difficulty is outlined further. Following this, various attempts to resolve the value conflicts are discussed. These possibilities are considered:

1. Finding some ultimate value or ultimate ordering of values.
2. Finding a set of rules.
3. Appealing to the law.
4. Settling for relativism.
5. Making an appeal to the relevant facts.

The Problem of Value

It should be clear that any answer to the problems raised in the case studies must involve some reference to values. For instance, if it is felt that Kathy, the health education officer who has been instructed to carry out a radical campaign against drug misuse, is right in her misgivings, then this feeling may be based on reasoning about the practical consequences. But at some point subjective values must have a part to play. Perhaps it will be felt that Kathy should have more autonomy, or that the public has a right to be informed rather than frightened. These are value judgements.

The alternative view, that Kathy's misgivings are ill-conceived, will also rest ultimately upon values. Perhaps it will be thought that Kathy should conform to the wisdom of her more experienced superiors, and that any course of action is justified in order to eliminate drug abuse. How can a value conflict such as this ever be resolved? This chapter demonstrates one answer, but first it is necessary to clarify something of the nature of value.

What Are Values?

In moral philosophy 'value judgements' and 'value-laden statements' are sometimes discussed. What is meant by this terminology?

Different sorts of value

It is natural for human beings to think of some physical things as more valuable than others—a motor car might be more valuable (both in terms of its monetary value and its practical use) than a bar of chocolate—and human beings also think of less tangible things as being more valuable than others. For instance, most of us consider that happiness is to be valued above misery, that life is to be valued above death, that pain is not to be valued, that work and creativity are to be valued, that the owning of property is to be valued, that truth-telling is valuable, and that trying to help friends is important.

Distinguishing values

How can different types of value be clarified and distinguished from one another? How can this be done so that more light is thrown upon the nature of morality?

The analysis of values given here is by no means exhaustive. This is not one of the purposes of this book. However, it is important to note that (a) not all types of valuing have implications for ethics in either the 'dramatic' or 'persisting' senses, and (b) all valuing is done by a subject existing within a wider culture. Distinction (a) raises the question of what types of value are possible. Distinction (b) raises the issue of the source and formation of values.

(a) Not all types of valuing have implications for ethics in either the 'dramatic' or 'mundane' senses   If a person values a principle, for instance, 'the truth must always be told', then clearly this value can have implications for ethics in the 'dramatic' and 'persisting' senses. If a person values his own life, or values some personal property, and another person wishes to take these valued things away then this conflict of values is likely to raise a 'dramatic' ethical issue. However, if a person has an aesthetic value (for instance, if she values a picture or a poem) or another type of intangible value (perhaps she values a particular friendship) then the mere fact that the person holds this value does not raise this sort of ethical issue—although there will always be some implication for ethics in the general sense since this view of ethics takes comprehensive account of how a person chooses to live her own life. And what one values or chooses to value are fundamental features of a life.

Types of valuing   The following distinctions of types of valuing are not watertight. They overlap in significant ways. However, the distinctions serve an important clarifying role.
   A person can be said to have a value when he finds something—anything—valuable.

(i) It is possible to value physical things, such as compact disc players, money, and cats (unless those cats keep breaking teapots).

Does this type of valuing relate to morality?

The answer to this question is that this type of valuing (and all the other types listed) relate to morality in different ways dependent upon what is meant by morality, dependent upon which part of the iceberg is perceived to be most important at the time. Consider two items of property—your neighbour's house and a favourite talisman. If morality is thought of as merely a question of right and wrong, and certain 'moral rules' or commandments have been laid down to define what is right, then valuing property will be simply either right or wrong dependent on the context. For instance, if it is a 'moral rule' that it is wrong to covet another person's property, and you covet your neighbour's house, then valuing that physical thing is wrong. Yet if you value your own talisman, and there is no ruling about whether this is right or wrong, then valuing a physical thing is neither morally right nor wrong. Valuing this object in this context, according to this sense of morality, is a non-moral or ethically neutral valuing.

   However, observing a different section of the iceberg—taking morality to mean 'ethics in the general sense'—coveting your neighbour's house is not necessarily a moral wrong. For instance, this coveting, although not normally regarded as a positive emotion, might stimulate activity to change your own house, to create something worthwhile for yourself. And valuing a talisman might be enabling. It might provide emotional support through life, and as such it is a moral valuing in the general sense of morality.

(ii) It is possible to value objects for their aesthetic qualities. For instance, it is possible to value works of art and poetry. Again, whether or not this valuing relates to morality depends upon what is meant by morality.

(iii) It is possible to value *intangibles*, such as friendship, introspection, and creativity.

(iv) It is possible to value principles. Whether or not these should be described as moral principles depends on what these principles are, and on what is meant by morality. For example, one might value the principles that 'all life is sacred' and 'all people are entitled to equal respect'.

   An important point about valuing principles is that it is necessary to reflect on these principles, to conceive of them, to arrive at judgements about whether or not they are consistent. This is an essential feature of moral reasoning.

   If a person holds principles that are in some way inconsistent then it is a task for philosophy to bring them to the surface, to make the inconsistency apparent, in order that the person might develop her personal reasoning further. For example, if a person holds the principle that 'all life is sacred' and so is absolutely opposed to vivisection, yet also believes that in order to protect national sovereignty (another personally held fundamental principle) it is right to go to war, then he is being inconsistent and must decide which principle is basic so as to overcome this inconsistency.

(v) It is possible to value ideologies, such as patriotism, or liberalism, or fascism.

(b) All valuing is an activity done by a subject within a culture   All human beings capable of intellectual reflection will have some value or other. It is possible that some of these values may be innate. They may arise out of a genetic imperative; for instance, people value their own lives. But any attempt to list 'innate' values will be fraught with controversy. What is clear is that some values depend upon the culture and era in which the subject exists. For instance, valuing paid work is only possible if such an institution exists. This sort of value can be fostered (Thompson 1985).

This raises an important question over the source and formation of values, and the source and formation of morality. There is a difference between human values and morality. These differences depend upon which senses of value and morality are in play. Given this, it is worthwhile to ask which notion—human value or human morality—is basic. Or whether at this level there is no difference between value and morality.

Morality or value—which is basic?

Options:

(i) It is possible that cultural values *create* all moral principles and all moral reasoning. So all morality rests on human values which stem from culture. Whichever values currently predominate in a particular culture, these are the source of what are taken to be moral principles. So if 'social stability' is a fundamental value then all moral principles will be defined in such a way as to ensure that social stability persists.

(ii) It is possible that cultural values are independent of morality.

(iii) It is possible that cultural values and morality are partially separate and partially dependent. (This is the option advocated in this book.)

(iv) It is possible that moral reasoning and moral principles create cultural values, that morality is basic. It is possible that an objective morality can be universally apprehended: that there is a touchstone that creates values.

Consolidation

In this section a definite link between human value and morality has been established, although the precise nature of this link must remain an issue. Since it can be demonstrated that values are an inevitable part of health work then this is further evidence of the depth of the moral content of the work.

Values Permeate All Health Work

It can be tempting to think that work for health is value-free, that some endeavours are simply good and desired by all, and have no effects that can be described as bad or undesirable. How can there be any quesion that curing diseases and mending broken legs is good?

In many situations and contexts health work should be described as good, but not in all. Is it moral to attempt to cure pneumonia in a patient who is suffering the final stages of terminal cancer? Is it moral to perform a hip-replacement operation on a 90 year old suffering from senile dementia? Is it moral to allocate the scarce resource of kidney dialysis on the basis of predicted life years? Is it moral to mend the broken leg of a man condemned to be executed the following day?

There are specific choices that have to be made in everyday practice, there are choices of ward policy in hospitals (should severely handicapped children be saved by heroic medicine, or should they be allowed to die quietly and with dignity?), and there are choices which concern the whole shape and organization of the health service: which priorities should receive funding—heart transplants, or cures for acne, or disease prevention campaigns?

It is an inescapable truth that all work for health, every last bit of it, is at some point inspired by a human value that has been chosen from alternatives. This sets the decision over what the health service should be doing, what it should look like, not in an unassailable objective position, but firmly on the shoulders of those people with the power to change it. All health workers are included in this number even though in most cases the power to create the new paradigm is not direct.

Even advice to exercise is not value-free

Why pick exercise as an example?   The reason for selecting the example of exercise is that it is commonly regarded as an activity that is good, something that anyone who is fit enough ought to do because then he will be fitter still. Some people even go so far as to argue that people have a duty—to other people and to the State—to exercise, since by exercising they stand a better chance of avoiding disease and illness that might adversely affect other people in some way, and would cause an avoidable financial burden on the State.

A view that advice to exercise is value-neutral   'Surely everybody knows that exercise is good for you. Surely, then, it must be true that well-intentioned advice to exercise "sensibly" must be a good that everyone will agree about. Advice to exercise, then, is objectively good advice, and as such it should be considered to be value-free.'

But it is not value-free. The mistake is to believe that what you like is what everybody else likes, or at least ought to like 'if only they knew what was good for them'. And to believe that this preference must hold true universally. This mistake should be condemned because it underrates the opinions, knowledge, attitudes, and experiences of other people.

The following discussion is not intended to convey the impression that there is no practical and moral difference between exercising conscientiously and smoking 40 cigarettes a day on public transport. All advice does not depend solely on subjective value. There is an objective element (for instance, the effects on the body of exercise and smoking can be measured), but even advice to exercise is problematic for the following reasons:

(a) There is no agreed definition of fitness   The goal of exercise is fitness. However, there is no agreed definition of 'fitness'. It does not appear to be possible to offer a universal standard of fitness because people have different physiques, and are of varying ages and of one of two sexes. The actual goal for individuals—that they choose to call 'fitness'—will always to some extent depend on subjective opinions about the nature of 'fitness'. For instance, the decision about whether stamina, suppleness, muscle development, or some combination of these factors, is of prime importance for personal fitness can be informed by detailed measurement and investigation, but must ultimately depend upon subjective judgement.

Fitness and convention   Further to the above point: the actual goal of 'fitness' aimed for will be influenced to some degree by prevailing social trends. To an extent the idea of 'fitness' will depend on the body shapes that are fashionable, the sorts of physiques needed for labour, and trends in preventive medicine and 'health education'.

So, a statement that 'Andy has optimum physical fitness' will rest partly on measurement and comparison of statistics, and partly on human definition and social trends.

(b) Advice to exercise can lead to undesirable consequences   Not everybody wants to exercise. Some people find the activity boring, tiring, painful, and a waste of time. Constant advice to exercise might conceivably force people into doing something, perhaps trying jogging, that is against their real wishes. And if people consistently refuse to exercise despite continuing well-meaning pressure the advice to exercise could create guilt and stress, and unnecessary anxiety about what damage not exercising might be doing to their bodies.

There are significant risks associated with exercise   With all forms of exercise there are well-documented risks (Katch and McArdle 1983) of injury and even death. Advice to exercise will not in all cases lead to desired ends. This calls into question the view that advice to exercise always promotes a 'good'.

An illustration of the extent to which values permeate health work interventions: the health visitor, the doting daughter, and the *Sporting Life*

Carole, a health visitor in the Handsworth area of Birmingham, UK, has been assigned an elderly lady called Veronica, who lives with her daughter Maggie. Carole has worked in the area for just over three months. She is 25 and, despite her demanding job, still rather shy and reserved. Carole's parents have lived in Harborne (a prosperous area of Birmingham) for 23 years, and Carole has not yet left home, although she did commute during the period of her nurse training. Carole reads the *Daily Mail*, always dresses 'smartly and sensibly', and could be classified as 'lower middle class' (both her parents are primary school teachers). Carole hopes to move from Handsworth to a more rural 'patch'.

Veronica and Maggie, the family Carole has to visit, live in a Victorian terraced house which has been divided into two flats by their landlord. They have a feud with the couple who occupy the other flat, who they say do not keep their three Alsatian dogs quiet enough. Veronica's condition has prompted the visit since she has recently had a urinary infection, and her doctor thinks it appropriate to keep a friendly eye on her progress. Veronica is in her mid-seventies, and, when Carole arrived, was sitting quietly in her armchair, slim with grey hair tied back in a neat pony tail, and with the grace and elegance that sometimes accompanies age borne stoically (*). Maggie, the daughter, in great contrast, is short, less than 5 feet tall, and very fat, almost comically round with huge owl spectacles. She is in her early thirties.

Carole spoke to Veronica, who tried to reply but was repeatedly interrupted by the ebullient Maggie. It was established eventually that the urinary infection and sporadic incontinence had improved markedly, and was no longer of concern. Instead Maggie seemed almost obsessed by the urge to have her mother fitted with a hearing aid. Maggie's argument was that her mother had difficulty hearing some television programmes, although she clearly had no trouble catching what Maggie and Carole were saying to her. Veronica steadfastly refused to try a hearing aid. She said she didn't want to be a nuisance, and she didn't need one anyway. Carole noticed with regret that Maggie treated Veronica as if she were a little girl, despite her still impressive appearance (*).

Maggie was loquacious on the topic of herself and her mother. She informed Carole that both she and Veronica were dependent on the State for their income (*). They had six cats, all of which were content and well fed (*). Maggie was bubbling with news of her mother's recent medical history, and of her own career at the surgery. She seemed proud that she too was to pay a visit to the doctors that evening. It seemed to the health visitor that Maggie's *raison d'être*, her motivation, was her mother (*), and Carole thought that this was rather a shame because Maggie was certainly intelligent and articulate.

The living room in which the consultation took place was unquestionably grimy. It had not been washed or dusted for months, it seemed. It smelt musty, and slightly of stale sweat and stale food. The room was generally untidy and, although only small for a living room, it contained an enormous electric fire, and two equally intimidating television sets, one on either side of the fire. It was three o'clock in the afternoon. By making her visit Carole had obviously interrupted Maggie during a meal since she could see, on top of a cluttered sideboard, a plate stacked high with chips, gravy, sausage, baked beans, and lamb chops. Carole could not help thinking that this sort of meal was really the last thing that Maggie wanted in her obese state (*). And what was worse in Carole's eyes was that most of the papers which littered the room seemed to be recent copies of the *Sporting Life* (*), the paper for people who like to gamble on horse racing. The latest edition rested on the arm of a soft chair—obviously Maggie's—placed only 3 feet away from one television (*). The chair was supplemented by an array of greasy cushions, and a portable trolley stood by its side.

Carole waited for an opportunity to leave. She thought she might hasten her departure by offering to take Veronica's pulse. Maggie accepted this proposal—on condition that she had her pulse taken as well. Carole was relieved that she could at last do something vaguely medical so that she could truly say that she had visited the family to further their health.

As she left, Carole reflected that she would be very depressed if she had to live a life like that in conditions like those. At the very least she would have made the effort to redecorate in pastel shades immediately.

Comment   There is a minefield of values and value judgements present in this example. The most obvious areas in which they might arise have been indicated like this (*). There is valuing of relationships (Maggie and Veronica), valuing of aesthetics (the appearance of Veronica, the appearance of the room), valuing of lifestyle (the horse racing hobby), valuing of cleanliness, valuing of personal lifestyle (the 'health risk' of obesity and overeating), and valuing of technique (the medical intervention when the pulse was taken). On top of these values there are examples of specific moral judgements—judgements about what is right and what is wrong—where the three people are in conflict. For instance, Carole believes that Maggie is morally wrong to treat her mother as she does (Carole also believes that Maggie is morally wrong to *treat* herself as she does) yet Maggie believes that she is justified in her actions. Not only are such statements as 'Maggie is a bad daughter' value-laden, but also far less overtly judgemental statements such as 'Maggie is overweight', 'Maggie eats unwholesome food' and 'Maggie's house is a mess' have a subjective content.

In this example many of the value judgements that are being made are reasonably clear to outside observers even though they are not so apparent to those who are directly involved. These value judgements do not occur only in the context of professional health work interventions, or only between people who come from different class backgrounds. On the contrary, value judgements are made in all encounters, even those where people share the same values.

It is vital that health workers become more accomplished at recognizing the varieties of values that are in play. Many disputes and much bad feeling over 'moral issues' comes about simply because the alternative values are not recognized as alternatives. Each side in a debate tends to regard their own position and outlook as right, and that of the 'opposition' wrong. Whereas, if the values are actually spelled out and clarified it becomes far easier to see the situation from alternative perspectives (Is Carole *totally* correct in her view? Is Maggie truly wrong—isn't she happy? Is she morally wrong?) It also becomes a lot easier to try to win the other person round to your way of seeing things because it becomes possible to discover a route into a different way of thinking, to recognize what another person holds to be important.

'Evangelicism'—A False Start

Certain people can best be described as 'moral evangelists'. Such people attempt to solve the problem that there is a proliferation of conflicting values in two inadequate ways: (a) by resort to rhetoric rather than reason, and (b) by appeal to a single value, or set of values, as the only possibility. The slogan is always that there is no alternative.

An example

In 1986 there was a well-publicized controversy about the rights of parents to be informed by general practitioners if an under-age daughter requests contraception (the legal age for consent to sexual intercourse in the UK is sixteen). The issue hinged on the question of whether or not the consent of the parent should be necessary. Mrs Victoria Gillick, a self-appointed 'campaigner for parents' rights', desired to retain and protect the total authority of parents over their offspring. Her position—which she stated to be the only morally acceptable position—was that sexual intercourse under the age of consent is not desirable. From this point she went on to insist that anything that encourages this (for instance, the prescription of contraceptives) must be bad, regardless of any other good that might be done (for instance, a reduction in teenage pregnancy.)

Mrs Gillick is a good example of an advocate of morality in the 'evangelical' sense. 'Moral evangelists' do not belong exclusively to right-wing political groups. There are many of left-wing persuasion who are just as doggedly single-minded. For example, the Labour MP Clare Short introduced a Bill to outlaw the publication of pictures of topless women in newspapers. She argued that such pictures exploit women and encourage male violence against women. Her argument has merits, but it is not the only point of view that can receive moral justification. Against Ms Short it may be argued that such censorship constitutes an unacceptable lowering in the level of civil liberty in Britain.

'Moral evangelists', whatever their particular point of view, picture controversies as stunningly clear-cut. There is always one single position on the controversy that is correct (i.e. their own position) while every alternative is wrong, usually to exactly the same degree. For such 'evangelists' morality can be understood only in the 'dramatic' sense. They are able to see only the tip of the iceberg, and because of this they can be frustrating opponents in debate. It is often tempting to conclude that such 'evangelists' hardly touch the moral issues at all.

Can These Conflicts be Resolved in a More Satisfactory Way?

There are five possible routes towards the resolution of value conflict, five paths to take in the search for what is truly moral.

1. Finding some ultimate value or ultimate ordering of values—the quest for objective morality

The discussion that follows is not meant to imply that a degree of objectivity is impossible in moral reasoning, merely that it is difficult to discover the correct path towards this level of objectivity.

It is a common belief that what is 'morally good' must be an 'objective good'. That is, if an act is said to be 'morally good' then this judgements rests on something more than opinion. There are some acts that are simply good, and that any sane human being would agree are good. It follows that statements about 'morally good' acts are objective, and that if a number of these statements are combined it is possible to have an objective system of morality.

Thus it can, on the face of it, appear that some statements are unquestionably morally correct. These examples are prime candidates:

'The absolute truth should be told at all times.'

'It is a moral obligation that professional duties should be performed to the best of the professional's ability.'

'The guiding principle of health work is never to do anybody any harm.'

'At all times the health worker's role is to encourage the maximum possible autonomy in the lives of all the people she deals with.'

Ways of analysis

These statements have been selected for analysis because they are among the most commonly seen moral principles in medicine and health studies. By careful analysis it is possible to show that these statements are not unequivocal but controversial. This shows that the appearance of objectivity that they convey with authority is actually deceptive. This calls into question the notion that there are actions and beliefs that can be described as simply objectively morally good.

There are at least three ways of analysing statements and combinations of statements of this sort.

Way One   First, *the apparent maxims can be examined individually in the abstract.* For instance, is it clear that a health worker should tell the truth in all cases? Further issues need to be considered. For example, it is not always clear what the truth is. In many circumstances it is difficult to be certain what the facts are; for example, which writer on nutrition should the health worker refer to for his advice to the client?

It has been argued that there is a difference between 'telling the whole truth' and 'giving a client a true picture'. Much health work involves specialist knowledge, and Western medicine is based on the study of complicated scientific disciplines. To tell the client 'the whole truth' about a particular condition, to explain the biochemistry, the physiology, and the histories of like conditions in other people, might not be feasible. There may be little time and a proper understanding might require prior knowledge in the client. Consequently, the most pertinent points have to be selected by the health worker. It will be her opinion that the client has a 'true picture', but this opinion will not necessarily be shared by a different health worker, even from a similar background.

A further complication may arise in that it might be the opinion of the health worker that the person is obnoxious and idle. For the health worker to tell the whole truth this would mean telling the client her true opinion about him, and this might not be the best way of encouraging his recovery or autonomy. Further uncertainty can occur if the health worker has factual information that might be detrimental to the client, or that the health worker is holding in confidence. For instance, the health worker might be aware that a client's wife is seeing another man. This is a significant factor in explaining the wife's recent offhand behaviour, which is depressing the husband and causing him to smoke more heavily than usual. The husband has come to the health worker for help in stopping the habit. The information held by the health worker is both true and relevant to the client's health concern, but should the truth be told? In what sense would the husband be enabled if he were to learn this information from the health professional?

Way Two   The second route of analysis is this. *The maxims can be applied to specific practical situations in order to see how they might work out.* Consider the apparently moral statement, 'At all times the role of a health worker is to encourage the maximum possible autonomy in the lives of the people he deals with.' It is not difficult to imagine real situations in which the maxim is, at best, uncertain. Imagine that you are introduced by a friend (who is aware that you are a health professional) to an acquaintance of his who has been taking a range of drugs and now wants to move on to heroin, but is uncertain about the safest way to inject himself. He has read about the drug and the risks and argues that he has made an autonomous choice to experiment with heroin. As a health professional do you encourage him in his autonomous decision (perhaps even injecting the heroin for him) or do you inform the police? If you justify a decision to tell the police by arguing that this will ultimately encourage the drug taker's autonomy in the future (i.e. once he is no longer able to use drugs he will eventually have a wider range of opportunities to choose from) you will still have acted against the apparent maxim (and there is no certainty that a drugs conviction will not close more doors to the person than would be the case if he continued with his habit). Another topical example might concern a health worker who knows that a man carries the AIDS virus and has continued to take sexual partners without informing them of his condition. How is this man's autonomy, his freedom to direct his own life how he wishes, to be encouraged without the health worker acting to debilitate the autonomy of his unsuspecting sexual partners?

Way Three   *A third way of analysis is to study these apparently objectively moral maxims in the light of the available range of ethical theories.* Knowledge of these theories mitigates against the tendency to make sweeping statements without taking time to reflect more carefully about the issues. The statements themselves can be assessed within the context of a particular ethical theory, in order to see whether that theory would entertain the spirit of the statement, or whether it would be part of a refutation of the statement. For instance, a utilitarian health professional might take issue with the statement, 'The guiding principle of health work is not to do anybody any harm.' The utilitarian might say that in many cases it is right to harm a few people in order to ensure the maximum possible (aggregative) benefit for the remainder. For example, a hard-headed utilitarian might argue that the British Government should take immediate steps to quarantine for an indefinite period any person known to have the AIDS virus, that every member of the population should be screened for the virus, and that any visitor to the country should also be screened and not permitted entry if he or she is a carrier. (If these examples seem difficult to resolve it is suggested that they be considered afresh after Chapter 10 has been read.)

From these three ways of analysis it should be clear that it is far from easy, and might not be possible at all, to define what is 'morally good' or 'objectively moral'.

2. Finding a set of rules—the quest for a binding moral code

An opinion exists that inquiry in ethics is nothing more than a matter of finding the set of moral rules which ought to govern human behaviour. The idea is that once the right rules have been uncovered and accepted there will be no ethical dilemmas that cannot be resolved, and all the erroneous theories can be discarded. But this point of view is mistaken. Ethics is not a science, it is not an activity that can be properly pursued merely by following rules. Most moral philosophers throughout history have agreed that ethics has a connection with rules and rule-following, but only a few of these thinkers argue that the generation of universal rules is the ultimate aim of moral philosophy. A genuine part of inquiry in ethics is aimed at the creation or discovery of ways of acting that, if well formulated and consistently followed, can help guide human conduct in ways that are agreed to be desirable, but this is not the complete story. It is a misperception to think that the aim of moral philosophy is to come up with a set of principles—some sort of Midas formula—that will always give the right answers, that will always turn a hard dilemma into a golden solution. Instead, the realistic aim of ethical inquiry is to clarify the issues, to show those who have to make decisions the full range of possibilities open to them, and to explain different perspectives and ways of reasoning.

The trouble with the point of view that ethics is only a question of finding the right rules is that there are no rules that can cope with all possible life situations. There are no moral principles that can be applied appropriately across the spectrum of human experience. No moral rule exists that cannot be broken with justification in certain contexts. For example, if the moral rule is 'never murder' (where murder is by definition the intentional killing of another human being) then it appears at first sight to be a universal rule. It was once legal in Britain to take the life of a convicted murderer in retribution for his crime. But now it is not. Such retribution is itself now defined as murder. This shows that rules and definitions are *created by human beings*, which substantially detracts from the claim to objectivity.

Further, there are a significant number of people in Britain (probably the majority of people) who regard the legally condoned act of retribution—legal execution—now defined in law as murder to be morally acceptable. These people do not regard the present legal rule—and the purportedly universal moral rule, 'never murder'—to be the best possible moral option.

As a further example, decisions are made and actions taken in medicine to let people die when their lives could have been prolonged by certain techniques. Arguably these actions constitute illegal killing with intent: murder. Such actions are at least manslaughter. When it is felt that it is better for a person to die rather than be maintained through artificial means—perhaps the person is old, comatose, and not considered to have a chance of ever again being autonomous—treatment is discontinued. And it is discontinued in the knowledge that this action will eventually result in a death that could have been avoided, although for reasons that can be justified, for exmaple, on the ground of respect for human dignity. On such occasions the 'moral rule' 'never murder' is, at least, called into question.

Rules of games and rules in ethics are not synonymous

In competitive games, such as cricket and football, binding and absolute rules are essential. Without rules to give the game its structure and organization there would be no game. The rules of cricket and football have been developed to a high degree of complexity in order that they will be capable of controlling every possible situation that might arise during the course of a game. It is a prerequisite of participation in the game that players agree to every rule. If they then transgress each player must accept whatever punishment is laid down in the laws. In competitive games it is usual to have an independent judge (an umpire in cricket and a referee in football) whose role it is to make sure that the rules are followed. The independent judge is an essential element of the game, but he does not participate in it as a player.

Games are artificial. They have been created by people who have defined the exact limits of each type of game. A game is like a world apart. Within the game rules are absolute, and whilst the game is in progress there can be no outside interference with the rules. It follows that games are qualitatively different from life in the real world, which is not only vastly more complicated, but, crucially, not enclosed by unbreakable rules acting to define it. Human beings create moral rules, just as we invent rules for games, but unlike games these moral rules are cast in very general terms, and are not specific to certain contexts as are rules for games.

For example, one popular 'moral rule' can be summed up by the dictum 'Never kill another human being'. This rule asserts that it is wrong, in any circumstances, to take the life of another human being. However, it is possible to imagine particular situations in which obeying this rule would bring about a greater evil than breaking it. For instance, it can be argued that it is morally better to shoot dead a deranged man who is holding 150 people hostage on a plane and threatening to blow them all to pieces, than it is to do nothing in the hope that he is bluffing.

Rules can be very useful guidelines which can, if adopted, provide a basis for daily behaviour. But it is essential to remember that there are many situations which might occur in which rules are unable to advise an appropriate course of action. Professional codes of practice are a good example of this phenomenon.

Codes of practice usually lay down general principles but they cannot advise the professional on the best interpretation of the principles, or inform her about how to decide between principles which conflict in practice, or how to decide when it is most ethical to disregard the rules and deliberate instead as a unique and independent individual. The following examples of rules taken from current codes of ethics show, without the need for any further comment the extent to which they have to be interpreted in context:

- Any act or advice which could weaken physical or mental resistance of a human being may be used only in his interest. (BMA 1984, p. 58)

- A doctor must always bear in mind the obligation of preserving human life. (BMA 1984, p. 59)

- Members will use appropriately their professional skills in the fulfilment of health education/promotion activities which they believe to be effective. (The Society of Health Education Officers, Code of Conduct, Principle of Practice 2)

- A doctor must preserve secrecy on all he knows. There are five exceptions to this general principle:

  (1) The patient gives consent
  (2) When it is undesirable on medical grounds to seek a patient's consent, but is in the patient's own interest that confidentiality should be broken
  (3) The doctor's overriding duty to society
  (4) For the purposes of medical research, when approved by a local clinical research ethical committee, or in the case of the National Cancer Registry by the chairman of the BMA's Central Ethical Committee or his nominee
  (5) When the information is required by due legal process (BMA 1984, p.12)

- Members will use their professional judgement regarding the confidentiality of information to which they have access, bearing in mind the requirements of the law and the best interests of their clients. (Ibid, Principle 10)

What is becoming clear is that what health professionals need are not only codes of practice (and a certain amount of knowledge of law) but in addition (and more importantly) a wider knowledge of ethical theory and modes of moral reasoning in order that they can refer to rules, if this is appropriate, but are also able to practise moral deliberation and apply personal judgement.

The problem can be summarized in this way:

(a) If the rules or codes are cast in very general terms then they will either be open to interpretation (e.g. 'practitioners should always uphold the highest professional standards') or there will be specific cases which contradict them, where there is a need for exceptional action (for instance, there are occasionally good reasons that can be advanced for the breaking of confidences). In such cases morality can be increased by breaking the rules.
(b) If the rules are specific, if they are addressed to certain contexts, then it is inevitable that future specific cases will occur for which no rules have been given.

Even if both general and specific rules are prescribed problems (a) and (b) persist.

Rules should not be ignored in health work ethics

It is possible to imagine a continuum of positions on rule-following. At one extreme there is dogmatic and consistent rule-following, and at the other arbitrary personal choice. Neither of these poles should be considered to be satisfactory if health work is to achieve the highest degree of morality.

Personal choosing by health workers, made entirely without guidance about rules of conduct, is not a workable policy. Health workers need the assurance provided by rules, and it is necessary to have a degree of consistency to ensure public confidence. A further practical point is that health workers are legally accountable for their actions and would be reluctant to do anything without the support of rules, without the rules being in existence to shoulder a large part of the responsibility.

However, it is equally essential that any code of practice or set of ethical principles is never considered absolutely binding. It is neither desirable nor possible to design a set of principles which will spoon-feed health workers with the right moral decisions. Most sets of principles are written in terms so general that they are open to a very wide range of interpretations. And if they are written as specific context based prescriptions they will fail to encompass the range of tasks and interventions done by health workers.

Summary

The benefits of having rules and following them are: (a) if rules have been drawn up and agreed then it is likely that these rules will be based upon reasoning and analysis; (b) the rules will provide useful guides for action; (c) the rules will be public—those who are dealt with by health workers will be able to know the rules; and (d) the rules will be universally applicable.

The disadvantages of always conforming to rules are: (a) people's powers of judgement and autonomous decision-making tend to atrophy if they are not used and explored. These powers will not be used if all that a person has to do is to follow a number of

principles in all possible circumstances; (b) whatever the moral rules prescribed exceptions will always occur where breaking a rule will produce a higher degree of morality
than abiding by it; and (c) a defining element of moral deliberation about how best to
act is that there must be uncertainty, at least at first, and that there must be a choice
possible. To state beforehand that whatever the circumstances a particular principle will
be upheld is to negate morality. Without the possibility of choice moral deliberation is
sterile.

3. Appealing to the law—the quest for moral legislation

Legality and morality—a tangled web

It is important to show that it is possible to distinguish between legality and morality.
One reason why the legislative bodies of professional organizations recommend codes
of practice to their members is that there are many types of human conduct which are
potentially harmful but which do not break any law (for instance, publishing information
that was given in confidence). It is argued that such conduct is unethical (in the sense
that it is wrong rather than right) but not illegal.

Often the sorts of behaviour defined as legal in a society will also be the sorts of behaviour that are generally described as moral. Equally, illegal actions are often thought
to be immoral. However, these are not the only possible classifications. It is enlightening
to try to untangle a web which surrounds this issue. By doing this it becomes possible
to arrive at a more complete understanding of what ethics is.

Clarification by separation

Note: laws vary between nations and societies. This is a further complication. Unless it
is stated otherwise the laws referred to in this section are based on current English law.
Yet a further complication arises from the fact that what is considered to be moral and
immoral can change dependent upon what sense of morality is in play.

It is possible to make six basic distinctions, all of which can be illustrated with examples. Acts may be judged to be:

(a) **Legal and moral**   There are many examples of this category. For instance, it is legal
and apparently moral to donate money to charity, to work voluntarily with disabled
people, or to listen to another person as he relates his troubles. Some 'moral actions'
are legally enforceable, although there is a question about whether actions done under
duress, that is not done freely of a person's own volition, can be said to be moral. For
example, courts of law compel witnesses to tell the truth as they know it. Legal contracts
are enforceable by law, which is an official way of ensuring that people keep promises.

(b) **Legal and immoral**   At this point ideas of morality can conflict with what is defined
as legal.

Consider the following examples: arguably all are immoral in some sense, and all are
legal under British law. Although these examples are highly contestable it should be
emphasized that it is necessary only to concede the possibility of any one example being
valid to recognize the sharpness of the distinction between legality and morality.

   (i) When a person breaks a marriage vow.

  (ii) When a person makes a promise without intending to keep it.

 (iii) When a lecturer offers higher grades to a student than his work merits in return for sex.

 (iv) When government ministers cut the money available to higher education, and consequently deprive some people of education they could otherwise have benefited from.

  (v) When a soldier kills a person in war.

 (vi) When a person is imprisoned purely as a punishment, without attempt at education and rehabilitation.

(vii) When governments or other powerful organizations deprive certain groups of people of rights that are enjoyed by other groups, and which could be permitted to them also. One current example of this can be seen in South Africa.

(viii) When people legally intentionally physically or mentally injure or disable other people. For example, it is legal in some Arab states to cut off a hand or both hands of a person found guilty of stealing. As a further example, the possession of cannabis resin carries a mandatory death sentence on conviction under Malaysian law.

(c) Illegal and immoral   There are many apparently clear examples of these acts. For example, it is illegal to commit robbery, as it is to commit murder, and there is a strong argument that these acts are also immoral.

(d) Illegal and moral   Like the combination of legal and immoral, this category can provoke much debate. In some cases, although not all, what is legal and what is illegal is clear. However, when considering whether illegal actions can be said to be moral it is necessary first to specify the sense in which 'moral' is being used. This requirement draws attention to the ambiguity of much ethics. Very few moral issues are in sharp focus as either black or white. Most are covered by different depths of shadow.

Consider the following examples. Arguably all are moral in some sense, and yet are illegal under British law:

   (i) When a person breaks a speed limit in a car in order to drive a man suffering from a heart attack to hospital.

  (ii) When a group of people obstruct traffic in a city by a 'sit-down' demonstration against the presence of nuclear weapons in Britain.

 (iii) When a person embezzles money from a major industrial company in order to donate it to various children's charities.

 (iv) When a charitable organization breaks a country's import regulations in order to get life-saving food to starving people as quickly as possible.

  (v) When a person employed by the Department of Health and Social Security interviews a claimant with real need, and yet is prevented by a technicality from providing help. Nevertheless the employee falsifies certain of the claimant's details in order that the need can be met.

 (vi) When a general practitioner fills out a sickness certificate falsely in order to help the patient. For instance, it might be the case that the doctor is unable to find any specific complaint but believes that the patient would benefit from some time away from the pressures of work, and so she reports some very general condition—perhaps stress, depression, or viral illness.

(e) Legal and amoral   With this classification everything depends upon the sense of morality invoked. If the only sense of morality considered is that of ethics in the 'dramatic' sense, ethics at the tip of the iceberg, then there is much activity that can be described as 'legal and amoral' because so much activity is neither moral nor immoral. However, if morality is thought of in the 'general sense', where all activity or inactivity can have some moral content and consequence, then little or no activity can be described as 'legal and amoral'.

Arguably, hobbies such as gardening or painting, running to work rather than walking, walking only on the joins of pavement slabs, or sleeping, are activities that are 'legal and amoral'.

(f) Illegal and amoral   As with the 'legal and amoral' classification everything depends upon the sense of morality in play. However, it is possible to argue that according to some uses of 'moral' there are examples of actions that are 'illegal and amoral'.

If it is accepted that both intentions and consequences have to be taken into account when assessing the morality of actions, it can be argued that an illegal act which the

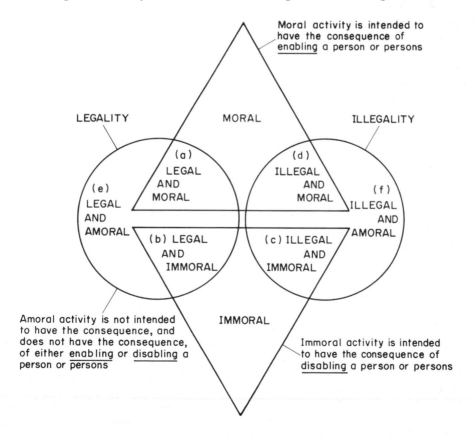

Figure 6   Distinguishing law and morality

offender did not *know* to be illegal can be neither moral nor immoral, and so must be described as amoral. For instance, a person might park his car illegally in a foreign city without wishing to break any law or realizing that he has done so, and without causing any other person any harm. Or a person might genuinely forget to have her car MOT'd (an annual test of roadworthiness which is a legal requirement in Britain) thus breaking the law, but not offending any moral standard (unless the view is taken that law sets the moral standard).

Figure 6 illustrates these points.

It can be easily seen that the quest to find the truly moral through legislation is doomed to failure. What is legal and what is moral are not necessarily the same things. There are some laws that are fundamentally immoral (see later in this chapter for the argument for this point). It may be that to ensure at least minimal levels of morality in a society a system of law is necessary, in order to maintain order. But this is not to say that any system of law is a truly moral system.

4. Settling for relativism—giving up the quest

So far it has been shown that it is not possible to discover a single objective value that can be said to be truly moral. Nor is it possible to invent rules, or laws, that when consistently followed will constantly produce the most moral outcomes. Consequently it might appear that the only solution is to adopt a relativist position. In this section this position is outlined, and its serious flaws are indicated.

The problem in general

In order to outline the idea of *relativism* it is helpful to contrast the position with an alternative position that might be called *objectivism*. Arguments between relativists and objectivists can be found in the philosophy of any discipline. The basic stances of each position are these.

Objectivism

There is a metre rule in Paris which is the standard to which all other metre lengths must correspond if they are to be called metres. This physical metre is the objective measure because all other lengths can be measured against it in order to see if they are metres or not. It is a standard of truth which permits the discovery of truth. Objectivism holds that in all other disciplines there are standards of truth that are exactly analogous to the metre rule, even if it is not yet clear what these standards are.

For example, in science it might be argued that the overall goal of scientists is to discover truth about reality. And further, that some scientific theories come closer to the standard of truth than other theories. For instance, it might be argued that in physics Relativity theory is more objectively true than Newtonian theory.

As far as societies are concerned it has been argued that various forms of societies can be judged to be more or less primitive in relation to how 'rational' they are. This view rests on the opinion that there is an objective standard of 'rationality' and logic which some of the human race have discovered. If some societies are found to behave in ways which seem unreasonable or illogical when judged by the standards of the anthropologists studying them (where it is assumed that the anthropologists are privy to the objective standard), then it is argued by objectivists that these societies are to some degree irrational because they do not conform to the true standard of rationality. Some anthropologists have studied 1987 post-election Britain in this light.

Relativism

Against objectivism, relativists insist that there are no objective standards of truth. As far as societies are concerned relativists argue that each social system will operate according to some standards that are not endorsed by other societies, even though many standards might be held in common. There are degrees of difference but if societies work according to their own standards and tenets then it is wrong to criticize them on the ground of 'irrationality'. Some societies operate with different forms of rationality, logic, and truth. The anthropologist who assumes to judge an alien culture as 'irrational' or 'illogical' is not able to make this judgement according to an objective standard, but is able to do so only on the ground of his own cultural norms. For the relativist, if another society does not conform with the norms that the anthropologist calls rational then the other society is irrational only in the opinion of the anthropologist. Societies can be said to be irrational only when compared with standards found in different societies, but this does not mean that the society that is perceived as alien is truly irrational because there is simply no standard external to human societies by which to judge this. Standards of truth are relative to different contexts.

It is not difficult to see how these opposed positions can come into conflict in moral philosophy. The following examples have been selected to show this.

Types of moral relativism

All the following theories can, to different degrees, be described as relativist. None of these theories supports some ultimate standard of morality, and they draw much of their strength from denying the existence of such a standard.

Emotivism

This point of view was put forward by A.J. Ayer. At its simplest the theory states that the only difference between a statement describing facts, and a statement describing facts and also offering a judgement about the morality of the facts, is the personal opinion of the speaker. So the statement 'the nurse did not explain to the patient what the likely side-effect of his treatment was' is distinguished from the statement 'the nurse was wrong not to explain to the patient what the likely side-effect of his treatment was' not by a difference of truth or falsity but merely on the ground that the second statement has added words which express disapproval of the nurse's behaviour. This 'moral judgement' is a value judgement and, according to Ayer, it is not possible for people to contradict each other about statements of value because such statements have nothing to do with truth or falsity. There is simply no arguing about questions of value because they have no factual basis and so there is no way of testing to discover which judgement is best. Everything is a matter of opinion. All one can do is to continue to express one's opinions, to continue to give expression to one's emotions.

The emotivist position is that any apparently meaningful argument about an 'ethical issue' is never a genuine argument since ethical judgements are kinds of feelings only, based ultimately on the psychological state of each interested individual. All that can be said of each feeling, each emotion, each value is that each is of exactly equal merit—all the opinions are as good or as bad as each other; since there is no separate moral standard existing outside emotion and feeling there is no yardstick against which to measure the different opinions. This means that it is impossible to decide who is right in ethical disputes.

What is wrong with this theory?   The basic problem with this theory, as with all relativist theories, is that it provides no solid ground on which to stand. Relativist theories deny that it is possible to make moral judgements that can be said conclusively to be better than alternatives. 'Emotivism' asserts that to respond according to one's feelings is as proper and valid as to respond using reason.

Although it is true to assert that value judgements in themselves cannot conclusively be said to be true or false (just as it is not possible to say conclusively, so that everyone will be certain to agree, that a particular painting or record album is definitely good or bad), it is short-sighted to say that ethical disputes relate only to people's emotions or psychological states. While subjective opinion about an interpretation of issues is clearly an essential part of moral reflection, the real world (other people, the law, the risk, the effectiveness of interventions), and the outcome of decisions and actions in the real world, are an integral part of morality. There is more at stake than opinion and emotion. For example, although it might not be possible to reach agreement about value judgements it is often possible to discover which outcomes will most favourably affect the people involved.

Egotism

Egotism is more a simple assertion than a theory. Egotism is the view that equates being moral with the consistent pursuit of self-interest. The moral egotist asserts that what is morally good is dependent upon what is in his interest. The ethical egotist insists that the good is what is good for her. The theory does not claim that the achievement of the interests of other people are an equivalent moral good. A form of this theory has been a main theme in theoretical economics. The 'rational man' of the economist is the self-interested man, the man for whom altruism and respect for others as moral agents has little or no meaning. The 'rational man' takes other people into account only in so far as they are a threat and are in competition for the same scarce resources that he covets. If the idea of morality has any meaning at all for the economic theories which espouse 'rational man theory' it exists only in relation to egotism and the desires of the individual.

What is wrong with this theory?   The problem with arguing against versions of relativism is that since the existence of objective standards is denied the relativist has only to argue that his version is on a par with any alternative that might be offered. The tactic that has to be adopted against the relativist, without accepting the assertion that there can be no such thing as an objectively moral act, is to examine the fullest implications of the theory and to demand the fullest possible justifications for the premises of the theory. For instance, egotism might be shown to depend upon psychology and theories of altruism and genetics. If this is accepted by the egotist he becomes far more susceptible to argument and empirical test.

This is not the task of this book. Instead a positive argument is put forward that morality does have a real basis in fact. The ideas of morality and health are closely associated. What is certain is that most health workers will find the egotist account of morality alien since it stands opposed to the values implicit in the everyday care of other people. Egotism is also foreign to the view that moral activity is essentially a process of reflection and deliberation which takes account not only of the self but also of other people as equals—to each other and to the one who deliberates. This view of moral activity rests on the premise that, although people are not the same, we are all equal in some fundamental respects (see Chapter Six). Given this assumption it is possible to conclude that 'egotism' is not a theory of morality at all.

Cultural relativism

This form of relativism is mentioned here as an option less extreme than the previous two versions. In relation to morality, for the cultural relativist, the question of what is right and what wrong does not rest finally on the opinions or feelings of individuals. Instead, it is believed that a set of principles—or general notions about right and wrong—are generated by the social arrangement of different cultures. What is considered to be morally right and wrong is not just a question of individual whim and psychology but the result of a 'social agreement' that has arisen out of the custom or convention of a particular culture. But the objectivism goes no further than this since the cultural relativist argues that there is no standard of right or wrong beyond the standards of each culture. The ethical codes upheld in one culture might not be thought morally right in another, and there is no possibility of deciding which culture has the correct view. For example, it has been documented (Warnock 1971) that Eskimos believed it to be morally correct for children to kill their parents while they were still able-bodied, before they became senile and decrepit. The consensus of the British outlook is that such behaviour is clearly immoral: the idea of children putting their parents to death is abhorrent to many people (especially to parents). And it remains abhorrent even when the justification for the behaviour is understood. It was an Eskimo belief that in the after-life people retain the physical bodies they possessed at their death. Consequently it makes sense to kill people (with or without their consent) in order to ensure that they are not disabled in the next life. According to the cultural relativist, since there is no such thing as objective morality, there is no possibility of deciding which view—the Eskimo's or the average Briton's—is moral.

It is taken for granted by many citizens in British culture that the principles under which we have lived for generations are objectively good. For instance, 'democracy', 'free speech', freedom from fear of death at the hand of another, freedom to own property, and equality under the law, are all considered to be objectively moral principles. But this is challenged by the cultural relativist. She points out that the British people have not always held such values and may not hold them in the future; there are those who would change them because they do not regard them as the most moral possible. British morality is objective only in the sense that the majority of the people tacitly assent to it. This system is no more and no less moral than that of the Eskimo. They cannot be compared since there is no absolute or universal human morality.

All the above types of relativism, to different degrees, make the claim that the search for morality, at least for an external objective morality, is misguided. Paradoxically, relativist theories can inspire the search for a universal standard since there is a need not only to be able to give reasons why a certain practice can be said to be morally better than another, but to be able to justify these reasons with reference to an ultimate standard. Unless this is possible, unless some answer can be found to the relativist case, there can be no distinction between the statement 'you ought not to kill me because it would be immoral' and the statement 'you must not kill me because I do not want you to'. But there should be the world of difference between these two statements. The first implies that to kill a human being is wrong because it offends against a universal moral standard, while the second asserts that it is wrong to kill a human being only because that human being is interested in self-preservation.

Human beings have an indefinite range of interests, and these are frequently in conflict. What is needed is some standard or set of standards to provide some arbitration, some sort of moral guarantee, in cases where interests are in competition.

There is a plausible answer to the relativist. The answer lies in an appeal to the facts.

5. An appeal to the facts—the focus on what is

Before the path towards the truly moral is mapped out it is necessary to introduce an important distinction, a distinction between what is the case and what *ought to be* the case.

The distinction between 'ought' and 'is'

This distinction is introduced as a preliminary stage in an argument to pin down the source of morality. The distinction between 'ought' and 'is' shows clearly that the idea of morality has been at least partially created by human beings and our values. However, this truth does not necessarily imply that morality has no basis in reality. It does not follow that all ethics stems only from opinion.

The distinction between 'ought' and 'is' demonstrates that statements about morality are qualitatively different from statements of fact in that they can never be proven. However, statements of fact *can* sometimes be verified. Armed with the knowledge of this distinction it is possible to avoid the trap of confusing evidence of what is (fact) as evidence of what ought to be.

Consider the following statements:

Eric took £5 from his grandfather's wallet.

Ian took the gun and shot John three times between the eyes.

David donated £20 to Liveaid.

Anne told a lie in order to spare her boyfriend's feelings.

Although it might be agreed that each of these statements has a moral content, knowledge of the is/ought distinction makes it clear that the moral content is added by human beings. Without our opinions and impressions all these statements are only reports of facts (that is, so long as the statements are true). We might think that Eric was wrong to take £5 from his grandfather's wallet (if we assume that he was stealing it) but nowhere in the act itself, or in the statement reporting the act, is it possible to discover rightness or wrongness, an 'ought' or an 'ought not'.

Oughts—moral judgements—cannot be derived from what is. What is just is. This point is purely logical. It is not logically valid to argue from premises of fact to conclusions of morality. It is not logically correct to argue from what is to conclusions about principles and ethical rules. The moral element is smuggled in, in this fashion:

Ian took the gun and shot John three times between the eyes.

Killing people is morally wrong.

Therefore Ian was wrong to shoot John three times between the eyes.

The first premise is of a factual nature. It is open to empirical test of some sort. The second premise, 'killing people is morally wrong', is not factual. It is an opinion and not open to empirical test.

How does awareness of this issue add to this inquiry into the ethics of health?

It is important in these ways. First, it helps to reinforce the point that there is no objective morality to be discovered in the sense that Mount Everest exists to be discovered. Human beings cannot embark on empirical field trips in order to find out what is truly right, it is necessary to use reason to reflect on what is best. In a real sense it is the human race which invents the 'ought'—morality is not independent of us, we create it, at least partially.

Secondly, the is/ought distinction can make us wary of arguing that because the group of human beings of which we are a part acts now in a certain way, because the group is as it is, this is the moral—or the most moral—way to behave.

But most important of all we can now begin to understand that, although moral judgement has been shown to have an essentially subjective nature, this does not mean that it is impossible to base moral principles in something objective. Although it is logically incorrect to derive an 'ought' from an 'is' as described above, it is not invalid to base a theory of what is morally good on certain matters of fact. How can this be so?

The moral quality of actions depends at least in part upon the value of what they bring about. In order to know whether some action is morally good it is necessary to understand what is worthwhile in a factual sense, and to know whether or not the action is intended to promote what is good in this sense. Taking the ideas of work for health and moral endeavour as being as one, it is possible to focus on the encouragement of human potential as being a valuable good that is based on fact. Work for health is work to enable biological and physical human potentials, and moral endeavour is work to promote the good in this sense too. Health work interventions are intended to liberate factual human potentials.

This insight undermines the is/ought objection. Being human and possessing a range of potentials is a fact which *contains* an ought. The statement 'Fred is a human being' contains within itself, implicitly, the statement 'Fred ought to be a human being'. This cannot be denied without absurdity. What is questionable, however, is the precise nature of what it is to be human. This book contends that practical work for health and the theory that lies behind it make explicit the reasons it is valuable to be human, why we human beings value our lives. And it is this which unites the ideas of health and morality.

This argument cannot be made quickly or easily. The following section is intended to provide further support for the position that the base of morality rests in human nature and potential. If it is true that morality cannot be discovered as an objective entity, as if it were Mount Everest, and if it is true that there are no moral goods or rights beyond human value and thought, the impetus must be to examine what is of central importance to human beings, what human beings have in common, what human beings are *for*.

A Search for Immorality: Grand Thiam

Discovering the nature of morality by focusing first of all on its opposite: immorality

As is demonstrated in this book there is a baffling variety of candidates for the title of 'the good', for the description 'truly moral theory', and for the ascription 'right'. And there are no uncontroversial criteria for judging between them. Because of this it is both sensible and legitimate to attempt to distinguish which type of action is truly immoral, in order to see what new light is cast upon its polar opposite—the moral.

An example from social work

This process is common in social work. In case conferences there is frequently a wide divergence of opinion about what constitutes a 'good parent'. For instance, is a good parent a person who truly loves the child but sometimes leaves it unattended for long periods? Or is a good parent a person who has little feeling for the child, who perhaps resents the presence of the child, yet who still provides diligently for the material necessities of the child's upbringing? Or is a good parent a person who has such deep love for the child that she will never let him out of her sight? Which parent comes closest to being the ideally good parent?

What is important in the context of this inquiry into ethics and health is that although there is inevitable and endless controversy about the definition of a 'good parent' it is possible to reach universal agreement about what a bad parent is. For example, all social workers agree that a bad parent—whatever redeeming qualities she might have—is a person who consistently and deliberately inflicts physical and mental harm upon her child, without ever reflecting on what might be good for the child, and without ever intending to produce a later end result which will enhance the life of the child.

On the Objectively Immoral: Grand Thiam

The following hypothetical society is described for two main reasons. First, it is offered as a clear example of immorality. And secondly, it is given to draw further attention to the very close association between the ideas of health and liberty. If the illustration is felt to be too abstract and fanciful it can be made more relevant by thinking about the *theme* of Grand Thiam in relation to real families, or in the context of familiar relationships between people, or with reference to politics and actions in the workplace, or with reference to a society which is either unable or unwilling to provide fulfilling work for many of its members.

The way of things in Grand Thiam

In Grand Thiam (a human civilization which has either existed in the past or will exist in the future—it does not matter which) medical technology has 'progressed' to the extent that it is possible to 'engineer' people in order to control them in various ways. One of these means of control is to inhibit them both physically and mentally.

At one stage in the history of Grand Thiam a momentous decision was taken by the ruling oligarchy (a group of 100 'Elders' who select their own successors in order to retain continuity of decision-making). This decision was taken in response to concern that the population of Grand Thiam was becoming increasingly rebellious and recalcitrant, despite its great prosperity. Even though the population had great material wealth many of their number were becoming vociferous: demanding power, demanding more liberty, and demanding the right to decide their own destinies. The Elders believed that a major contributory factor in what they saw as collective petulance was the policy of permitting higher education for all.

From the point of view of the Elders this pressure for change was a serious threat to their particular social priorities. For the Elders the ideal society is one in which there is strong social cohesion, where every member knows his or her place and is satisfied with it, where there is unquestioning obedience to the law, where all industry (whatever its nature) is able to achieve maximum productivity, and where disease is kept to the absolute minimum. This set of values is revered above alternatives, which might include principles such as continuing liberal education throughout life, free and uncensored speech, public participation in decision-making, and equal opportunity of access to power. Values such as these are thought to be highly dangerous and debilitating. The Elders' argument is that the more they proliferate the more social stability is threatened.

Dwarfing   Through a recently developed cocktail of medical and educational techniques it became possible for the Elders to engineer their ideal society. Part of the process made use of the Platonic 'noble lie'. All existing history books were destroyed and replaced by texts which indoctrinated the belief that a caste system is the only possible system on which an orderly society can be based. This propaganda was reinforced by techniques of genetic engineering, and the continuing addition of chemicals to the water supply. The intention was to alter the mental states and attitudes of the consumers. The Elders' aim was to ensure the creation and then perpetuation of their version of the 'ideal state' through restricting the very existences, in various ways, of the human beings who made up the society. That is, the aim was to limit '*the what might be*' to a '*what we say should be*'.

The implementation of the plan   The plan was implemented, in the early years, by weakening and numbing the curiosity, the power of logic, and the questioning power of the population, through the use of a range of drugs universally administered, and by radically increasing the banality of television programmes and newspapers. Then, as the population who had experienced relatively unfettered thought died off, the rate of the genetic and social engineering process was increased, so that all new members of the society could be fitted from birth, physically and intellectually, for their allotted roles (which were defined by a sub-committee of a working party of the Elders). The implementation of this process not only meant that people's intellectual powers were reduced and clouded (through lies, through indoctrination, through operations on the brain at birth, and through the use of drugs to which all members of the society were exposed) but also that the physiques of some of the population were reduced and limited artificially. The implementation of the plan made it necessary to interfere with the physical development of children in order to suit them physically, as well as mentally, for the tasks they were to take on in 'adult' life. This meant that for some jobs, such as the inspection of gas pipes, some types of mining, and the inspection of sewers, the physical development of some children was halted before puberty, and their intellectual development and 'knowledge base' (i.e. the amount of information that could be taken in) were restricted according to the complexity of the task they were to perform (if this seems too far-fetched it is salutary to remember the not uncommon practice in India for parents to cripple and mutilate one of their offspring in order to enable him to beg more successfully). In other words many children were intentionally deprived of the fulfilment of their natural physical and mental potentials to become adult. They were disabled and prevented from becoming fully adult persons in the interest of the society as a whole, as this interest was perceived by the Elders. These children were *dwarfed* deliberately.

A Major Connection

There is something which we know intuitively to be disgraceful and uncontroversially immoral about the process of dwarfing. The hypothetical example of the way in which people are treated in Grand Thiam makes a startling connection and implication crystal clear.

Health work is work against dwarfing

Examination of the theory and practice of health work shows that the underlying sense of health and work for health is the concern to remove or prevent obstacles to individual human physical and mental growth and development. Health work strives to enable people to bring to fruition the range of potentials that lie latent within them. By educating, by curing disease, by mending broken wrists, by developing personal power to conceive—to picture one's situation and future possibilities more clearly—*health work is simply the direct opposite of dwarfing*. As the exact counter-balance of dwarfing or 'the immoral', it follows that health work is objectively a moral endeavour. But since there are different types of health work, different senses of moral, and an indefinite range of contexts and ways in which it can be carried out, it is a mistake to assume that each task for health will be as moral as any other work for health. Just as in the two scenarios involving the young footballer with a broken wrist there are degrees to which the enabling (or anti-dwarfing) can be carried out, and different levels of moral intervention are possible. However, if the intent of the health worker is to enable the enhancing potentials of the person she is working with, if the path she pursues is one which she can justify with integrity, then the work will inevitably be moral. How close to the optimum degree of morality the intervention comes will never be absolutely certain, but will depend on a full assessment of intent, outcome, how far the intervention is in tune with basic tenets of health, and how far it is effective in the context of everyday life.

In the ailing paradigm of work for health there is a great imbalance between the attention given to the physical and that which is given to all other aspects of individuals, even though it is quite clear that the subject matter of genuine work for health is not just bodies but whole people, and the external factors and conditions which make up their lives. Work for health is comprehensive construction and maintenance of the foundations on which people can achieve. Very few honest health workers would take seriously the view that the end point of their health work is a non-diseased body. It is commonly recognized that health work does not strive to keep people alive as an end in itself—it does not work only on bodies and treat people as objects; instead the reason why bodies are given therapy is in order that the person may go on making real as much of his potential as possible.

Work for health can legitimately and properly be so much more than medical and hospital care, and traditional health education. For instance, it is presently uncontroversial in health work that children's eyes should be checked at an early age. The only debate is about how early this should be. Many health authorities recommend that children should have had their eyes checked by the age of three and a half years, but some specialists believe that this could be too late to remedy certain defects.

This example gives an indication of why the great imbalance has come about. Defects of vision can be detected and tested objectively, and something practical might be done about a problem to immediate effect. However, there is in principle no reason why a person whose intellect has stagnated at 36 as a result of a tedious job and unchallenging existence should not be equally a target for a health intervention. A person's intellect is just as much a part of him as his eyes, and its flourishing is arguably even more important if he is to become a mature and interested person. The problem in health work is that the values, political judgement, and empirical evidence involved with intervening with intellectual development are far more obvious, and the options are more contentious, than is the case with work with eyes, and other physical interventions. But just because this is a *difficulty* does not mean that the work is not genuinely part of the endeavour to create more health. In many medical consultations, in conversations between nurses and patients, in some types of health education, in women's health groups and neighbourhood schemes this endeavour is already going on. The extra that is needed in order to bring about the best version of the new paradigm is for the health service to acknowledge the width of health work in its rationale, and to make clear the inescapable conclusion that work for health—within certain legal and moral limits is work to liberate the fullest possible spectrum of human potential.

An objection

It might be argued that although the above account gives a correct view of the nature of health, it misunderstands the nature of potential. Since human bodies develop throughout life it is clear that there are always biological potentials that can be enabled.

However, this is not so clear in the case of intellectual potentials. For instance, school-ing stops at the age of sixteen because only a minority of people have the potential for higher education, just as it is a fact that only a small minority of people can become athletes or cricketers.

Against this objection it can be said that the assumption that only physical potentials continue to develop throughout life is based on poor empirical evidence. For example, work in psychology and psychiatry and in educational theory shows clearly the range of intellectual potentials that can be enabled throughout life. This evidence reveals further that development in logic and reasoning skills can be impeded or dwarfed through lack of practice, lack of expertise, and lack of the relevant information.

In short, the problem is this: we have, as a society, no difficulty in accepting that a working-class child's broken leg should be set so that it will develop as it would have if it had not been injured. This is clearly a task that can be tackled by a health care professional. What is more is that physical obstacles of this sort are not dealt with for their own sake. They are dealt with not only to restore normative biological functioning, but also so that a person can go on to live a fulfilled existence which he finds valuable. People are not put back on their feet for the sake of it, but in order that they can do more and be more satisfied. Physical potentials are enabled in order that enhancing mental potentials will also be liberated (Seedhouse 1986, pp. 72–5, for a discussion of enhancing potentials).

However, although the following strategies have a genuine theoretical claim to be described as health work, it is apparently more difficult to accept (1) that the same child's intellect should be encouraged to develop as it would have if it had been given the educational opportunities at home and at school that the most privileged children in a society have, or (2) that the same child's emotional development should be encouraged to continue as it would have if a broken marriage had not disabled it, or (3) that the same child's ability and opportunity to choose throughout life should be encouraged to flourish fully—this requires attention to the social conditions in which the child exists. For example, the opportunity to choose depends upon the extent to which information is available to a person.

Work for health is work directed against the intentional or accidental dwarfing of people. Since every aspect of a person's being can be dwarfed, work for health should be correspondingly comprehensive. As this conclusion dawns, and as the complex le-gal and ethical implications are recognized and confronted, so the new paradigm will crystallize.

Summary

In this chapter a number of possible paths towards the discovery of the truly moral have been discussed and rejected. What remains is the knowledge that it is necessary to consider human nature and potential, empirically, in order to understand better what human beings are for. Although it is impossible to give an objective list of enhancing potentials, and it is not possible to define what is truly moral, it is possible to be clear about what is immoral. This, and the implicit notion of dwarfing, are vital clues.

The following points are clear:

1. It has to be accepted that there is no such thing as 'morality' which has an existence independent of human beings. What would such a morality be like? The claims of some religious groups that ethical rules have been established by a supernatural entity are opinion only and cannot be tested. If one believes that a deity creates morality then everything is evidence for this, and if one chooses to disbelieve this claim then nothing counts as evidence for this. Crucially, since there is no evidence that would sway a neutral to believe that a deity creates morality the view cannot be sustained. It follows that the only possible place to search for an objective morality is in the human race. Given that there is no morality to be found external to human beings it follows that there is no ground for human rights outside human existence.

2. Given the merit of the arguments of the relativists it is necessary to accept that any opinion of any human being about what is moral and what is not will always be challengeable. It is always possible to advance viable alternative options. This is simply part of the diversity of human thinking. Because of this inevitable and legitimate diversity it is not enough even to search for common opinions shared by all human beings. It is not possible to discover values about which all human beings will agree. Not even seeking to avoid pain, seeking to avoid death, and valuing one's own life can be said always to be universal human values. For instance, athletes seek pain in order to push themselves towards higher performances, and people sometimes commit suicide. However, since these basic values will normally be shared they form a part of the story about morality.

The basis of morality

3. It is thus necessary to base the fundamentals of morality in the fact of human existence, in what is naturally human, without falling into the trap of mistaking an 'ought' for an 'is'. It is at this point that the notion of health can clearly be seen as central to ethics. The key is the fact that human beings do have certain physiological and mental potentials that are common to us all, and if these were not allowed to develop in some minds and bodies then these could not be considered to be full persons. The point is this. It is necessary to ask 'What is a human being for?' Just as the answer to the question 'What is a football for?' is a list of potentials and intended uses, so the answer to the question 'What is a human being for?' is a list of potentials. Some of these potentials, the very potentials on which health work concentrates, are essential to being a person. In the jargon, they are essential to minimal personhood (see Chapter Six).

4. Resting on the base of the three preceding stages and the idea that it is the achievement of human potential that is central both to health and to morality in the richest sense (the sense that takes in the complete iceberg), it is possible to develop the argument of this book that the fullest degree of morality, or of ethical intervention, is that which enables persons equally, without discrimination, to achieve the fullest enhancing potentials of which they are capable.

But more substance needs to be added to this theoretical analysis. In order to be more clear about practical and moral priorities in work for health it is vital to have an understanding about what people—or 'persons' in more technical language—are.

Chapter Six
What is a Person?

Introduction

As with other 'what is?' questions about complex notions and objects, the question 'What is a person?' is at once simple and yet perplexingly difficult to answer. The question 'What is a person?' might be answered simply by saying that 'a person is a human being like you and me', and this answer will be partially correct—but it is not the whole story. The question 'What is a person?' generates an indefinite amount of other questions, only a few of which can be tackled by the present investigation. What is needed is a plausible working definition of a person—to enable the understanding of precisely what the beings are that we consider so important and aim to equip with health, and what it is about persons that makes them so special. This definition has, of necessity, to be abstract, but this does not preclude empirical statements about specific nature and specific personal potentials. What is needed is a definition of 'personhood' that is not dependent upon particular cultures, periods in history, or ideologies, or on biochemical or psychological terms. The task of arriving at a definition of a person is a challenge for the enterprise of philosophical clarification. And although the definition of a 'person' must be cast in abstraction it is at the same time a task which can have real practical implications—for instance, a decision about whether or not to switch off a life support machine can hang on what working definition of personhood has been chosen. The decision will not depend only on this definition, but if it is finally considered that the body being maintained has no prospect of ever regaining the essential characteristics of 'personhood'—that, for instance, the body will never again be aware of itself—then this will at least be a significant factor.

Some Answers

To provide the discussion of this chapter with shape the complementary arguments of John Harris and John Dewey are outlined and considered. This analysis produces working definitions of 'person' and 'full person'.

The Argument of John Harris: Towards a Working Definition of Basic 'Personhood'

Harris (1985) begins his definition of 'personhood' by stating that the description 'person' points to certain features that make the existence of whatever it is that possesses them *valuable*. Like many other philosophers before him Harris uses the term 'person' in a technical sense, not just according to the ordinary meaning and use of the word—

which is to indicate a human being of either sex and any age after infancy. Harris argues that it is not strictly necessary to be human to possess valuable features (there may be 'persons' on other planets but these would certainly not be human beings like us), and that it does not follow automatically that being human means that the human body is definitely also a 'person' in the technical sense.

Harris goes on to quote an idea put forward by John Locke, an idea which Harris sees as an important forerunner to his own definition. Locke was concerned to pinpoint the essential features that distinguish 'persons' from other creatures, and also to help explain why we value 'persons' so much. The reasons that Locke advances help show how it makes sense, according to the richest meaning of health, to have a health service which enables persons rather than only bodies:

> We must consider what 'person' stands for; which, I think is a thinking intelligent being, that has reason and reflection, and can consider itself, the same thinking thing, in different times and places; which it does only by that consciousness which is inseparable from thinking and seems to me essential to it; it being impossible for anyone to perceive that he does perceive. (Locke 1964, Book II, Chapter 27)

Locke's point is that although it is not possible for a person to 'perceive that he does perceive' in terms of seeing or learning—one cannot see oneself seeing—a person can be aware of himself thinking.

Locke indicates a condition that is taken by many philosophers as being essential to the state of being a person: self-consciousness—the awareness of a reasoning process—that which enables an individual to 'consider itself, the same thinking thing, in different times and places'. Harris agrees that this is an essential condition but wishes to expand the idea further. For Harris another essential defining characteristic of a person is contained within the idea of *valuing*. According to Harris, for a human being to be classed as a person it has to have the capacity to value its own life. The above two conditions unite in this way: self-consciousness is necessary because in order for a being to value (or to have the capacity to value) its own life it has to be aware that it has a life to value. Harris's simple definition of a 'person' is 'any being capable of valuing its own existence' (Harris 1985, p. 18).

'Persons' and 'full human beings'

In his account Harris considers an objection to his position offered by Mary Warnock who is opposed to the use of 'person'. Warnock objects to the use of 'person' on the grounds that it is confusing and could be used as a convenient 'smokescreen', permitting any action on a being so long as it can be established that the being in question is not actually a 'person'. Instead of 'person' Warnock prefers the term 'full human being'. For her it is membership of the human species that is the vital moral principle, while for Harris it is the capacity of a being—any being—to value its own existence. Harris prefers his version over Warnock's because it avoids the possibility of discrimination between species.

Both the terms 'person' and 'full human being' are meant to offer basic criteria of identification. Neither of these terms goes further to specify what a fulfilled human being—a 'full person'—might be, yet this is an important step in the construction of a philosophy of health.

To Be a 'Full Human Being', or to Have the Capacity to Value 'Oneself', Is Part of What Is Meant by Being a 'Full Person', but Is not the Whole Story

Harris and Warnock offer specialized analyses. They are concerned to lay down basic conditions for 'personhood'. Both philosophers recognize the necessity to define the essence of what it is to be a valuable living thing. Both (despite Harris's concession to science fiction) see the need to describe the importance of individual human existence in order to explain why it is fundamentally immoral to treat human beings (the vast majority of whom will always qualify as 'persons') as objects, or with no respect, and why it is immoral to discriminate between beings who are *equal* in such fundamental respects. What is so significant about criteria for 'personhood' is that the very properties which define and identify 'persons' must, by definition, be held *equally* by all 'persons' or 'full human beings'. In order to have a clear moral base for medical practice, scientific research, and health care, it is crucial to have a 'bottom line'—a definition of a valuable life which effectively prohibits immoral treatment of that life. In the absence of such guidelines a door will have been left open by the philosophers of the day to leave unfettered those who would ignore the equality of the human condition, and who would exploit people unjustly for ends which are not moral.

However, in the context of the argument of this book, it is necessary to go further than Harris and Warnock. The principle of equal respect for 'persons' (the term 'people' can be substituted if it is remembered that it is being used in a technical sense) is of central importance to health work and rests on the fact that certain features of human existence are shared equally by all human beings. And this should guarantee basic human rights that are part of the rationale of health. However, health work in its richest sense includes not only the imperative to treat people with equal respect and to serve needs before wants, but also the imperatives to create autonomy and respect autonomy. Consequently, this account, whilst accepting the basic criteria for what it is to be a 'person' from Locke and Harris, finds it necessary to build upon this foundation to construct a notion of 'full personhood' which recognizes these other imperatives.

The idea of 'personhood' with which Harris is dealing recognizes only very basic, essential features. If a being to be a 'person' needs only to be able to value his own existence and nothing more it is hard to imagine what such a being would be like. Other capacities are implied by Harris's definition, but they are not stated. Because of this it is necessary to develop the idea of 'full personhood'. When Harris defines the importance of human life he does so in the context of *medical* ethics, that is, the sort of ethics which is associated with black and white decisions—the hard life and death choices, the medical traumas. Harris has a single-minded approach. In the context of cases in medicine where some people attempt to justify choices which undermine the importance of individual human existence (for instance, it can be argued that babies with certain forms of handicap should not receive medical treatment, and that some elderly people should not be operated on because the operation would cost too much, or might rule out a younger patient) Harris's simple question is: What is it about each individual that is important—what is it that makes life valuable at all? His answer is set in terms which refer to a basic potential: individuals have the capacity to value their lives, and they value their lives because they know that their lives will hold future choices. To deny an individual who finds his life valuable is fundamentally wrong. And this is where the argument stops. Indeed this is as far as it is necessary to go with the argument for the purpose of helping those with power in medicine to make moral decisions according to Harris's conception of morality. But, and this point bears repeating until it gains wide acceptance, the ethics of medical work is part, but not the whole story, of the ethics of health. In order to consider properly the idea and ethics of health it is necessary to consider *what these future choices might be*. For Harris's purposes this is not really important—all that matters is that there are some rather than no choices for the individual in the future. What is *different* about the ethics of health work is that it is necessary in the majority of areas of legitimate work for health that the worker considers carefully, in the abstract and in context, the nature of those future choices she is trying to enable.

Potentials

It is at this point that it would be satisfying to be able to state which empirical potentials that are open to people are good, and so should be enabled by health workers, and which are bad. But this is not possible. Individuals value different ends, circumstances are varied, individuals are varied—so a comprehensive list cannot be given. What are available as a guide for health workers are the essential elements of health work rationale and a thoughtful assessment of realistic potentials (Seedhouse 1986).

When considering the idea of 'persons' in the context of health work in its richest sense an important distinction should be made. It is necessary to distinguish between (1) the notion of human potential in the abstract, and (2) specific human potentials. This distinction provides an important section of the platform on which the theory of health and ethics advanced in this book stands.

The notion of human potential considered in abstract terms

It is this notion which inspires the fundamental principle of 'personhood' which Harris argues should be an inviolate standard in medical ethics. Without needing to consider contexts, or to be specific about actual people, it is possible to say that all 'persons' and those with the capacity to be 'persons' (that is, almost the entire human race) must have certain potentials. Harris believes that 'the capacity of the being to value its own existence' is the most fundamental potential, but there are others. For instance, all 'persons' will have the capacity to think and reflect, and, without exception, all living human beings will have bodies with the potential to continue developing in some ways. All human beings age so it follows that all human beings have biological potential.

It can also be said in the abstract that certain of these mental and physical potentials will be considered more desirable than others. For instance, it is usually felt that to age without physical pain is preferable to ageing in pain. And it is usually believed to be better that a 'person' values his own life because he can see reason to look forward to future opportunities, rather than that a 'person' values his own life simply because that life exists.

Although it is infuriatingly difficult to state clearly which potentials should be considered to be good and which bad, the fact that all 'persons' have some aspects of their lives which they possess equally and in common with all other persons, makes possible a powerful claim. Although it is not clear to what degree interventions to enhance people's lives can be said to be moral, it is clear that to intervene to prohibit the achievement of these basic potentials in some people and not others is a case of *selective dwarfing*, and as such is simply immoral.

Specific human potentials

It is at this point that good practical work for health depends upon the empirical investigation of actual potentials in individuals. Taking into account the two following conditions—that *the achievement of a desired potential in an individual should not decrease the amount of future potentials open to that individual that might enhance her existence*, and that *the achievement of the desired potential should not be at the expense of avoidable dwarfing in other people*—it falls to the health worker to consider with the client which of a range of possible potentials should be made reality. Sometimes the decision will be relatively simple. For instance, if the patient has broken his leg then the prime consideration will be the restoration of the normal biological potentials of the leg and the patient. During the treatment and healing process it will be possible to make actual certain other potentials, dependent on the skill and vision of the health worker concerned. For instance, the patient's confidence, knowledge, and understanding might all be increased by appropriate kindness, empathy, and education.

In the care of terminal patients the selection of which potentials it is possible to enable will be less complicated since time is short, but this selection might well be more painful than in any other area of health work. Much will depend upon the choice of the patient (autonomy is a basic human potential which follows naturally from the possession of the capacity to value one's own life), and hard decisions might have to be made about the balance between the elimination of pain and the extent to which the patient is able to communicate with those he loves and who love him.

The most baffling choices for health workers who seek to enable real potentials in the people they care for, face those who deal with people who have a lot of life to come. Such people possess numerous potentials only some of which they will ever make reality. If the health workers are to work consistently, according to the rich rationale of health work, then they must take into account the range of physical and mental potentials present in their clients. Even if the complaint is a simple physical one the best health worker will also seek to explore the client's feelings and the future possibilities open to the client, viewing his life as a whole. If the client does not wish for this sort of intervention then the health worker should stop. However, in principle there is a responsibility incumbent on the health worker who recognizes that *work for health is a moral endeavour* to discover which parts of the person lie latent and could be made actual with beneficial effects. This is an empirical inquiry: Does the client need help with a housing problem? Does he need advice about where to find friends? Will he benefit from an opportunity to take some programme of education? Does he have a sporting ambition or talent which is not being expressed? Does he have a creative ability or interest which might be developed by appropriate training and opportunity?

It is only if an impoverished view of health work is held that these potentials are not considered to be 'proper health work'. Against people who take this limited view these questions should be asked: Why is it thought important to cure disease—is it so that the morbidity statistics can be improved, or is it in order that a person can go on to achieve in his life? How does it make sense to think that the physical aspects of human existence are the most important when the very features that mark off 'persons' from other beings are their capacities for reason, for conceiving intellectually, for valuing their own lives, and for their autonomous development?

Work for health is work to create 'full persons' in a sense which goes much further than Harris's basic idea of 'personhood' and Warnock's notion of a 'full human being'.

Dewey's Idea of Personal Growth as the Only True Moral End

The elegant work of John Dewey adds further substance to the above discussion. John Dewey was one of the few major philosophers in history to take a deep interest in education, which he saw as a central *raison d'être* of philosophy. He believed that, in the general senses of the words, 'morals' is 'education'. Both notions are inseparable from the idea of growth of a child. The end or purpose of the educational process is not something outside it: 'Growth itself is the only moral end' (Dewey 1920).

In Dewey's view people are best equipped to realize their individual capacities within a 'democratic society', because

> All social institutions have a meaning, a purpose. That purpose is to set free and develop *capacities* [my italics] of human individuals without respect to race, sex, class or economic status. And this is all one with saying that the test of their value is the extent to which they educate every individual into the full stature of his possibility. Democracy has many meanings, but if it has a moral meaning, it is found in resolving that the supreme test of all political institutions and industrial arrangements shall be the contribution they make to the all-round growth of every member of society. (Dewey 1920, p. 147)

Dewey makes an important and comprehensive statement in this passage. His words are general and idealistic, but no less valuable for that. His sentiment is entirely in keeping with the spirit of the argument of this book. To paraphrase: Dewey's argument is that in a democracy any social institution (whether it is work, or school, or the family, for instance) is only moral in so far as it is directed towards the growth, in every possible way, of each unique individual in that society, regardless of race, age, sex, class, or economic status. Any social institution is valuable in proportion to the degree in which it helps every individual, equally, to achieve his or her fullest possible potential, as comprehensively as possible. For Dewey a society is moral according to the extent to which it allows each individual member to flourish.

This noble aim is precisely what a true health service should aspire to. Interventions made in this spirit aimed at these goals have the most moral intent. Any 'health service' that sets its sights lower than this—for whatever reasons—is not a health service in the richest and most humane sense of the word. Any 'health service' which does not have the goal of encouraging the development of 'full persons' (Dewey's 'flourishing human beings') might exhibit a degree of morality but this will not be the fullest degree of morality possible. It will not be the best possible health service, and it will be part of a correspondingly less valuable society.

The argument rests on the belief that the single most important principle of a civilized society must be that it is designed so as to provide the same degree of enablement to each of its citizens, regardless of their personal fortune or abilities. This is much more than a question of semantics. A health service based on these ideals will not only attempt to solve problems of human physique, and will not only make use of the techniques of medicine. It will be a health service which will, in Dewey's words, 'set free and develop the capacities of human individuals without respect to race, sex, class, or economic status ... [and] educate every individual into the full stature of his possibility ... Only by being true to the full growth of all individuals who make it up, can society by any chance be true to itself' (Dewey 1920).

A difficulty

Once again the problem of discovering a set of values on which all can agree has appeared. It is probable that to those of a socialist or liberal persuasion Dewey's fine rhetoric sounds convincing. But it might well seem to be nothing more than mistaken words without substance to a person whose views are influenced most by the politics of the right wing. The question of which potentials should be enabled over other potentials is clearly a political issue. For instance, in a society motivated by ideas of liberalism and individualism it might appear to be both desirable and appropriate to enable the potential to be self-seeking in another person, who one wishes to see achieve a higher degree of health than she has at present. Whereas in a society based on some rationale of community or collectivism it might be neither desirable nor appropriate to enable the potential to be self-seeking in one in whom you are trying to create health.

The political aspect of health care

The discussion has turned to expose the heart of the difficulty over the meaning of health. Since the expression 'healthy' is so value-laden it follows that a system of health care cannot avoid being, if not a system of direct political control, at least a system which receives its guidance and motivation from the political environment in which it exists. It might be that the system of health care of a country can provide a mirror reflecting the morality or immorality of the political system in which it operates. Different possible versions of health care can be arranged along a spectrum of types. For example, at one end of the spectrum there might be a system of health care devoted solely to the prevention and elimination of disease and illness. Its only function will be to return bodies to such a state where they can again be economically productive, or to make sure that illness does not restrict their abilities to produce. Between the poles of the spectrum there might be a system of health care (perhaps rather like the one that exists in Britain at present) where people are treated as individuals in their own right, but only up to an imprecise and variable limit. At the other end of the spectrum the health care service might be based on the ideology which inspires Dewey, and might limit its resources only when the national budget has been exhausted.

Which of these types is most moral in the general sense of morality?

The following answer is given in a different form elsewhere in this book. It is restated here for the sake of clarity, and in order that the argument can be seen to be progressing coherently.

An answer

This answer refers to Grand Thiam which was offered as a hypothetical immoral society.

It was decided that universal agreement about what is objectively moral could not be reached because there were so many plausible candidates for the label 'the good', and because unique individuals in any of an infinite variety of contexts would not all value the same 'goods' to the same degree. And further, people frequently fail to agree that what one of them believes to be a moral good is actually a moral good from another person's point of view. It is just not possible to state specifically what is definitely moral, at the expense of the elimination of the plausible views of other people.

However, it was decided that what is truly immoral is the deliberate restriction of individual potential to a state that is less than adulthood. Since it seems fundamental that it is simply immoral to dwarf people physically so that their bodies remain permanently the size of children (what possible justification could be offered for such a practice?), so it is at least equally immoral to disable intentionally a person's ability to reason and to reach autonomous decisions without his consent since it is precisely this facility that is believed to distinguish human beings from animals—or persons from non-persons. Although it is not possible to go on from this position to state precisely what actions in life are moral, or more moral than others, it is possible to assert that the degree of morality achieved through interventions in life will be higher the more they are in opposition to the notion of dwarfing.

Summary

The following major points have been made in this chapter.

The term 'person' is a technical term used by philosophers to describe beings with certain qualities. One such quality is the ability of the being to value its life. The possession of this ability implies a basic degree of autonomy.

By definition the basic characteristics must be possessed by all persons. This shows that there is a basic equality amongst all who can be said to be 'persons'. If the civilizing principle of 'justice as fairness' (see pp. 109–12) is to be taken seriously, since there is such equality of basic characteristics in 'persons', then there is a clear implication of a primary duty to treat all persons equally.

'Persons' can be defined in terms of *basic characteristics*. However, it is enlightening and appropriate in the context of health work to think of 'persons' in broader terms, that is, to consider the defining characteristics of 'full persons'.

One of the basic characteristics of 'personhood' is to have the possibility of future development. Although the degree and type of future development possible to 'persons' varies enormously, in every 'person' there exists the possibility to become more of what he could be. The onus rests with health workers to recognize the basic equality of 'persons', and to strive to ensure—paying the fullest attention to the talents of the individual concerned, and to the context of the situation—the maximum flourishing of the 'full person'.

The system of health care best equipped to do this is the system at the opposite end of the continuum to the system devoted only to the elimination and prevention of disease and illness. *A system with the goal of the fullest possible individual human flourishing is the most moral system of care.*

Chapter Seven
Theories of Ethics

Health workers of all kinds should have a competence in ethical thinking. In order to develop such competence to the full it is necessary to understand the theories of moral philosophers, and also the various problems that have been encountered by these theorists.

Health workers need more than a willingness to 'do good', 'to do the right thing', or 'to be moral'. Health workers need tools to be ethical just as a doctor needs his stethoscope to sound a chest, or a surgeon needs to know the theory of blood pressure and wound healing. Health workers need to know the basic content of and difficulties with the various theories of ethics, and they need to be aware of the different principles for action that follow from the various theories. Just like the surgeon seeking to gain skill with his knife, health workers need time and experience in order to develop their ability to work with these tools. Health workers need to become accustomed to moral reasoning. For example, in order to arrive at a conclusion about which actions are morally preferable in any given context it is necessary to decide which principle or principles of action are most basic. Dependent on the circumstances, it can be that the priorities should change, and this can be disorienting to those people unaccustomed to moral reasoning.

Introduction to Ethical Theory

The essence of moral reasoning

The point of describing and discussing the theories of ethics outlined in this chapter is to display the richness of moral reasoning. Moral reasoning has been described as a prism (Emmet 1979) which can shine different lights onto issues. Which light is shone depends upon the person who is to reason, and the more theories of ethics that are understood the more options there are about which light to shine. The point of describing so many theories is to make it utterly clear that it is inadequate to select one theory and apply it consistently to every problem or dilemma. It can be argued that simply adhering single-mindedly to one theory is not what it is to be moral at all. It certainly is not a practice that should be described as 'moral reasoning'.

A respect for moral reasoning is a sign of maturity in a person. It is a significant mark of civilization. Moral reasoning is made possible by intellect, stamina, and patience. Moral reasoning can be strenuous but the process is immeasurably more valuable than single-minded rule-following, or a total reliance on intuition. It is clear that there are no specific rules that can always be applied to best effect in all situations. And it is apparent that a reliance on intuition is not sufficient. However well educated and well intentioned a person is there is no guarantee that she will automatically, on every occasion, be able to intuit what is right. Not only will there be numerous occasions where equally well-educated and well-intentioned people have different intuitions, but some moral dilemmas (for instance, the 'tragic choice' given on pp. 43–4) generate more than one justifiable choice. If these choices seem to be of equal merit then a person who relies on intuition will flounder. It will be obvious that a more comprehensive and careful deliberation will be necessary.

The person dedicated to moral reasoning recognizes that rules and principles are necessary, but that they can come into conflict in theory and in specific situations. Consequently, these principles must be analysed in context in order to see which are the most appropriate to bring to bear on the situation. It is most easy to see this if the structure of the situation is separated out into the key elements, and the range of alternatives is made apparent. The pros and cons of alternative courses of action must then be weighed up and balanced against one another. Whichever course is chosen must be justified in some way; usually either by an appeal to a principle appropriate to the context of the situation, or by an emphasis on the benefit of the expected outcome. The person dedicated to moral reasoning does not make entirely *ad hoc* decisions. She is concerned to make her decision with the knowledge of the results of decisions made in similar situations in the past, and to examine decisions in the light of later events.

In Chapter 9 an instrument designed to enhance moral reasoning is introduced as a guide. It incorporates all the elements described above, and is intended as a starting point for personal reflection. Before the instrument—the Ethical Grid—is presented it is essential to prepare the ground by reviewing some of the classic theories of moral philosophy. Many situations can be resolved and many interventions improved simply by knowing and applying a particular theory. The following theories of ethics are not offered as simple recipes for morality. It is not suggested that one theory should be selected according to taste and used on all future occasions. The theories are introduced as a means of enriching moral reasoning, in order to enhance moral activity.

The point is not to advocate a particular *theory* (which has been the tradition in recent moral philosophy, see Warnock 1978), but rather a *general way of thinking*. The idea is not to encourage moral specialists, who support only one viewpoint in ethics, but to promote morality as a *general capacity*.

A General Distinction

As introduced briefly earlier (see pp. 24–5), the central distinction in moral philosophy is striking. It is between *deontology* and *consequentialism*. That is, it is possible to make a straightforward separation between the view that the essence of morality depends upon a person acting according to certain given principles, which is his duty, and the view that the essence of morality rests upon a calculation of the benefits and disadvantages of the consequences of actions.

As the intricacies of moral philosophy unfold this distinction can appear to be blurred. For instance, some deontologists justify their position on the ground that the overall consequences of abiding by certain principles are of ultimate benefit. And some consequentialists have argued that it is a basic moral duty always to try to assess the consequences of actions. It is not necessary to delve into these depths, but it is important to indicate the basic standpoints of the different theories.

Deontology

(The word 'deontology' is derived from the Greek word *deon*. 'Deontology' means 'the study of duty'.)

Central to deontology is the idea that to be moral a person must perform her preordained duty. In its purest or most extreme form deontology holds that a person should always, without exception, perform certain duties whatever the consequences. The precise nature of these duties is, to an extent, a matter of opinion. There is not one principle or duty on which all deontologists will agree. A deontologist might decide to adopt a single overriding duty—for instance, she might advocate that promises should never be broken, or that all people should be treated as one would wish to be treated if in their position. Or she might have chosen to adopt a range of duties, all of which make moral claims on her in theory.

If the deontologist takes the latter course it will be necessary for her to decide which of her chosen duties are of supreme importance if the range of duties happen to conflict in context. For example, the deontologist might espouse the principle that *retributive justice* (that is, punishment for a perceived wrongdoing) should always be administered. And she might also adhere to the principle that it is a fundamental duty always to keep promises. It is not difficult to imagine a case which brings these principles into conflict.

For instance, the deontologist may have promised a youth that whatever he tells her about what is depressing him will be told in confidence. He then proceeds to tell the deontologist that he has stolen several items of jewellery from his mother, which he sold, spending the money on fruit machines in order to satisfy his addiction to gambling. On the one hand the deontologist has chosen the duty that promises should never be broken, and on the other that wrongdoing should always be punished. She has made a clear promise to the youth, and the youth has committed a crime for which he is liable to be punished. The deontologist then has to employ the facility of moral reasoning in order to decide which of her duties should take precedence in a case such as this. Yet once she does so she will have to consider factors which are not purely questions of duty—for example, she might consider which of her duties will result in the best consequence for the youth in the long run.

Deontological theories contrast with theories which take the practical world as a major consideration. Two examples of theories of this sort are teleological ethics (that is, the version of ethics which maintains that it is possible to decide what actions ought to be done from a study of the things in the world that are good in a factual sense—see Grand Thiam section) and utilitarian ethics (that is, the variety of consequentialism that maintains that a decision about what actions ought to be done can be derived from a calculation about which action will produce the most happiness for the greatest number of people). Against these sorts of theory, which have in common the position that morality depends in some way upon factors that can be discovered through empirical investigation, deontological theories argue that the discovery of what is moral is either never, or hardly ever, a matter for calculation or research into what actually is. On the contrary, a deontologist—dependent upon how pure a deontologist he is—will argue that either there are some obligations and actions that are right and good in themselves regardless of the consequences, or that although it is sensible and important to consider the consequences of actions there are nevertheless certain duties that are of supreme and abiding importance.

Deontologists argue that it is wrong to ignore these principles, even in order to bring about the most favourable consequences in the short term. If the standards are over-ruled then the trap door has been thrown wide open over a slide into contingency, into making responses merely according to what seems to be the right thing to do for the moment. And worse, if basic duties are shunned then it becomes more likely that some individuals will be able to justify selfishness in pseudo-moral language. And further, even if it appears to be better in the short term to break faith with these principles, the consequences will not be better in the long term.

Types of deontology

Act-deontology

Act-deontology is a puzzling and extreme version of deontology because the principles and duties for action are not defined beforehand. Because of this it is perhaps a little contrived to include this ethic in the deontology section. This has been done because it is usual practice in ethics texts. The theory is against rule-following in principle. Sartre and other existentialists can be described as act-deontologists because they place the focus of moral action not on rules or code books or generalities, but on informed human judgement in the particular context of each new situation. The assumption is that however much one situation might appear to resemble another each context is unique, and just as each actor in it is unique so each judgement about it will be unique. This is held to be so if for no other reason than that the person who is judging *now* will be different in so far as he will have had more experiences in life than he had when he made the previous decision. There are no standards other than the central tenet that everything in morality must rest upon the person who is to judge and to decide. Principles are not basic, although they can be considered; consequences are not basic although they can be taken into account. It is the one who is to judge that is basic. The overriding duty in act-deontology is the duty of a person to be true to herself.

The advantages of act-deontology   It is not recommended that act-deontology should become the guiding moral theory for health workers enmeshed in the professionalized, bureaucratic modern world. There must be overt rules and principles of conduct to guide professionals in complex organizations. But the emphasis of act-deontology on being true to oneself in situations where moral deliberation is necessary is an element of morality that should never be overlooked, even in the most professional organizations. The spirit of act-deontology is the spirit which inspires the Ethical Grid.

Act-deontology begins to draw attention to the following areas. First of all the theory points out that there are no rules and principles that can be applied to future cases on the grounds that they have always been moral in the past, since each new situation—

however similar it might appear to a past one—is unique. Because of this uniqueness surprising things might happen and unexpected factors might need to be taken into account. Consequently, it follows that in all interventions it is morally inadequate for the health worker to abide by rules and convention. Each situation will be uniquely alive and will require the fullest possible attention from the health professional. Simply to do what you have been told to do, or to carry out your work as if everything is routine, is to deny the importance both of yourself and of the people in whose lives you are intervening.

And secondly, the theory of act-deontology explodes a myth that a professional is somehow different from a non-professional. It is thought by some that to be a professional (i.e. to have a specialist body of knowledge and skills unique to one's vocation) means that one person, in a sense, almost becomes two people. That is, it can be believed that an individual at work has 'professional responsibility' and makes 'professional judgements', and that these responsibilities and judgements are different from those he has when he is at home or on holiday—when he is some other person. Act-deontology insists that a person should be true to himself in every situation in which he finds himself, and being a professional for a time is just one more situation in which this authenticity is necessary. There is always a choice that can be made between doing what one is contracted to do and doing what one thinks one ought to do—if the two courses of action are different.

The disadvantages of act-deontology   A major criticism of act-deontology is that it is highly impractical. How can a system of care, or any other system, be built on a philosophy that advocates making arbitrary decisions? While it is true that every situation in life must have some unique aspects (even if these are only those of time, place, and participants), this is by no means the same as saying that *everything* about each situation or intervention in life will be unique. It can come as a radical deflation to a person, whether he realizes it as a child, as an adolescent, or in adult life, or whether he has to re-learn it from time to time, that there is actually nothing special about his life other than his own evaluation that his life is special. The human condition is such that we are confronted with problems which are often horribly unique to our individual lives, but it is rare that one person suffers a trouble that has not been suffered before by many other of his fellow human beings.

To sum up, although it can be said that some aspects of situations and some aspects of individual lives will be unique, it is also true that many other aspects of situations and lives have common features about which it is possible to make generalizations. Because of this it is clearly practical to draw up some set of rules (which do not, however, have to be finally fixed and static) in order to deal with situations and make interventions as morally and consistently as possible. Such rules require a stronger coherence and *raison d'être* than is the case with rules of thumb.

Rule-deontology

Instead of insisting that a person's moral choosing depends on how she sees the intervention, and rests on honest personal judgement, a rule-deontologist asserts that a person's moral choosing should depend upon a rule or set of rules that should be followed without exception, regardless of the likely outcome. Rule-deontology asserts that the consequences of not acting according to abiding moral rules will, either in the short or the long term, be worse than any alternative.

The advantages of rule-deontology   The basic advantage of rule-deontology is that the actions of those who espouse rule-deontology will usually be predictable. In the health service at present there are a number of codes of practice, which could be described as a limited version of deontology. The principles contained in these codes are usually too general to allow the degree of predictability required by deontology. One possible direction that the health service might take could be to draw up more precise principles of practice that could be applied according to the general philosophy of rule-deontology. For instance, it might be the case that rules such as 'always tell the truth as you know it', 'always keep promises', and 'always respect other people as you would wish to be respected' could become generally recognized principles of practice.

The disadvantages of rule-deontology   The main problem with rule-deontology is this. If a single rule only is chosen as the principle of health work then there will inevitably be occasions where it would be better if that rule were broken. For instance, there are occasions (although perhaps only a few) where it is better if promises are not kept. The trouble with rule-deontology is that, since the occasions on which the basic rule should be ignored are infrequent and unusual, it is not possible for a rule-deontologist to give a rule or instruction about when and how this should be done.

And if a set of logically consistent rules is chosen, then although they might appear to fit together in theory, sooner or later the actual situation will reveal conflicts between them. Again, the trouble with rule-deontology is that it offers no guide for the health worker to choose between the rules that have been thrown into conflict. If the rule-deontologist ranks these rules in some order of priority in order to escape this problem, then the initial difficulty remains. That is, there will always be occasions on which it is better to ignore even the primary rule, and no guidance can be offered about when and how to do this.

Should the Health Service Operate According to God-given Rules?

It is important to think a little about the sorts of argument that people of religious faith might advance in favour of the proposition that the health service should be based on rules passed on by a deity.

A significant number of people base their personal ethics on 'God's law', which is taken as a fundamental moral code. At their simplest these personal ethics are based on the assumption that an action is right or moral if it has been commanded or approved by a divine being in some way, and an action is wrong if that being has forbidden it. The central difficulty for any ambition to base a health service on God-given moral principles is simply that different people understand 'God's law' to mean different things. Dependent upon which god one recognizes (and this is naturally a major hurdle for a health service based in a multi-religious society), or even dependent upon which sections from religious texts are chosen, different moral principles might be followed.

The problems here are similar to those encountered by rule-deontology. They are:

1. Which of the various laws that are said to be God-given in religious texts are truly from a deity? Which are most appropriate for a health service, and which deity will confirm this? And if all the laws must be said to be of equal merit, and all of equal validity, then which should be adopted by a health service?
2. If *all* the laws are adopted by health workers then, in the inevitable cases of conflict between these laws in both theory and practice, how can health workers resolve this conflict? There is no God-given law in existence which clearly and specifically enables health workers (or anyone else) to decide which law should be applied in which context.

There are many compassionate health workers who act, both at work and at other times, according to principles and ways of acting which they derive from their religious convictions. And there are other equally caring health workers who act on principles derived from other sources. Whatever the nature of the well-intentioned principles, they do not necessarily require a religious justification. They can equally well be supported by the sorts of moral philosophy described in this book, or by humanist principles. And further, a religious justification for rules for behaviour is impossible to sustain without all concerned having the faith that there is real substance to religious belief. Since not all health workers and clients have faith it is neither practical nor necessary to base a health service on God-given rules.

The Influence of Immanuel Kant on Ethical Thinking

Kant's theory of ethics is forthright in clearly placing duties above consequences. Kant took it as his task to construct an objective ethical theory which did not rest on the ability to calculate the consequences of actions, but instead had its source in human reason. Kant's idea was that certain principles of behaviour, certain duties, could be discovered by any rational human being because these principles are part of the human make-up.

According to Kant, certain principles and actions are simply moral in themselves. Certain things simply ought to be done by human beings. Certain principles are just. Consequentialist theories cause deontologists, such as Kant, considerable disquiet since although the prescriptions of consequentialists are frequently practical they can also be harshly unjust and unfair to some people. Consequentialist theories exclude the element of human *feeling* about what is right and wrong. During consequentialist analysis of situations human emotions and beliefs about what is intrinsically moral can be discarded in favour of cold calculation. And because of this, deontologists argue that such reasoning simply does not qualify as full ethical reflection and activity. Rather, Kant argued that there are certain duties incumbent upon all human beings because of our very nature.

The categorical imperative

The major feature of Kant's ethics is known as the 'categorical imperative'. Kant argued that this 'imperative' is divided up into a number of 'forms'. Each of these forms is a duty incumbent upon 'rational human beings'. Kant claimed that each rational human being will be able to see the certainty and necessity of these moral laws by use of his faculty of reason.

It is not essential for the purposes of this book to assess all the forms of the categorical imperative, or to give an account of Kant's attempted justification of his argument. However, in the context of the present inquiry it is very helpful to examine in some detail the extent of Kant's emphasis on duty over consequences. When the Ethical Grid is brought into play and used it is essential that the user recognizes the tension that frequently exists between the pull of duty and the weight that should be given to consequences. An understanding of Kant's moral philosophy provides the necessary appreciation of the requirement to pay deep attention to duty during moral deliberation.

For Kant the only true moral action is one which is generated by a pure motive. The truly moral person will do what ought to be done, not after weighing up the pros and cons of what is likely to happen to herself and others, but simply because of a prior duty to obey the categorical imperative or moral law. Kant wrote, 'To duty every other motive must give place, because duty is a condition of a will good in itself, whose worth transcends everything' (Metaphysics of Morals). The truly moral act is not influenced by self-interest, nor by any consideration of overall social benefit. The key to morality, for Kant, is that the person who is acting must do so out of the pure motive of doing her moral duty.

What is the essence of Kant's 'categorical imperative'?

The central principle of the 'categorical imperative' is one which is familiar to several movements, both religious and atheistic. It can be summed up in this way. Essentially Kant's moral theory rests on the belief that human beings are entitled to equal respect. Although it is quite obvious that people have different abilities and must find themselves in different and changing circumstances, we have a sufficient number of shared features to make it possible to draw the conclusion that 'we are all in the same boat'. Given this conclusion it follows that no moral person would act towards any other person in a way that he himself would not wish to be treated. This spirit is encapsulated in Kant's first formulation of the categorical imperative. This is, 'Act only on that maxim which you can at the same time will to be universal law.' In other words, act in a particular way only if you would wish that anybody else, in like circumstances, would act in this way. So, for example, before you deliberately say something hurtful to someone else out of malice, or before you steal that handbag, or before you decide that no one will know if you say that you've paid your coffee money at work and you really haven't, or before you do nothing when you could have done good, you must genuinely will that your action become a universal law.

The essential features of Kant's ethical theory can be presented, in a simplified form, in the following way. It can be divided into three parts. The first of these is the general dictum discussed briefly above, the second adds more substance to the imperative, and the third part fully unites the other two.

These parts can be simplified in this way:

1. If you wish to act morally act as if your action in each circumstance is to become law for everyone, yourself included, in the future.
2. If you wish to act morally always treat other human beings as 'ends in themselves' and never merely as 'means'.

What Kant meant by this is that it is always wrong to treat people as if they are objects—mere tools to be used to further your own ambitions and ends. It is always morally essential to recognize that all other people have ends of their own. They have emotions, hopes, and anxieties just as you do, and just as you wish to be respected, other people's feelings and aspirations should be respected equally. According to Kant it is fundamentally immoral to exploit a person without considering her *as a person*, as an 'end' in her own right.

3. If you wish to act morally always act as a member of a community where all the other members of that community are 'ends', just as you are.

Why did Kant choose these principles?

The three parts of Kant's ethical theory are discussed in turn.

1. Kant chose this principle because of his belief that all people are entitled to equal respect. Kant recognized that it is a natural instinct (i.e. a reaction not based upon reason) for people to be self-interested (unless they have been enlightened by the 'moral law') and to weight whatever actions they perform in their own best interests.

   The idea that inspires the first principle is that an essential feature of morality is impartiality in the subject. If a person always operates according to the first principle it becomes fundamentally wrong for that person to make an exception of himself. In other words, when considering how to act it is immoral to believe yourself to be of any more merit than any other human being.

   The first principle does not specifically state which sorts of action are good or bad. But what it does do is to force the individual actor to examine her moral conscience every time she contemplates an action. If she decides that she would not like what she is intending to do to someone else to happen to her, or if she will enjoy what she is doing for herself but would not welcome the consequences if everyone else behaved in that way, then according to this principle she must decide that the proposed action is morally wrong.

2. This principle—always treat people as 'ends', not merely as means—is intended to add substance to the first. It is intended to provide a standard by which to assess whether an action is right or wrong. Kant was not so idealistic as to hope that in each everyday dealing we have with any other persons we will always consider their wishes and their goals. It would seem strange if we were to inquire into the life history of a shop assistant when we knew we were to meet with each other only once, and then only to buy a pair of trousers from her. In this case, or in the case of an employer and employee where the relationship depends upon a financial contract, it is inevitable that people (both the buyer and the seller, the employer and the employee) will treat each other and will be treated as means. For Kant there is nothing wrong with treating a person as a means provided that the person is not treated only as a means. To be moral in an interaction you must, whenever this is appropriate, also respect the other person's ends.

   To treat a person 'as an end' is to recognize that the person has his own purposes, just as you have yours. The secret is to imagine your own death. Imagine how much will be lost when you die—a lifetime of hopes, fears, achievements, and failure will disappear. A complete world will expire. Think of other people in those terms and you will understand what is meant by the advice to treat other people as 'ends', as other worlds.

Although the content of other people's desires and choices may be different from your own, you share the fact that you have desires and choices. To treat a person as an end rather than as a means is to act towards that other person's desires and choices just as if they were your own. So, if possible, you should work to fulfil the other person's wishes, so to enable him to make successful choices, just as you wish to make successful choices.

A clear example of moral wrongness according to this theory is slavery. When a person is enslaved he is, to quote Aristotle, treated as nothing more than a living tool. A further classic case occurs between some men and women where one totally dominates the other without considering that the one who is being dominated has the power, albeit latent in the circumstances, to decide her own destiny for herself.

3. The idea behind the third principle is that a moral agent should act always as a member of a community of persons, all of whom are just as able as the agent himself to make moral decisions. The implication of this, and the link with the other two principles, is that each member of the community will respect the desires of others and will allow them freedom of decision. They will recognize that everyone can and should decide and behave as if they, as a result of their choices and actions, are legislating for all.

The intent of Kant's philosophy is to argue that other people are just as competent as oneself to make moral decisions, and are entitled to the same opportunity as anyone else to make those decisions. This implies a real equality for all members of the human community.

Politics and ethics

Certain political conclusions follow from Kant's ethical theories. This close association between ethics and politics is not always recognized, but political implications inevitably ensue from any coherent theory of ethics which seeks to be prescriptive. The theory of ethics implicit within the Ethical Grid is just such a theory, and so has political consequences for health work and the health service. This theory, like Kant's ethics, can be described as an ethics of democracy, taking 'democratic society' as one in which every one of its members should have a say in how it develops. Kantian ethics also requires liberty, since each member of a society should be as free as possible to choose for herself, and it requires fraternity in the sense that each member of the community should consider himself a member of a moral community—a member of a community shared by others with equal moral rights and equal moral responsibilities.

Some Problems with Kant's Theory of Ethics

There is a major theoretical and practical difficulty with Kant's central doctrine: 'Act only on that maxim which you can at the same time will to be universal law.' The doctrine is intended to cause people to stop and think before acting. For example, a person who wished to be moral of Kant's sense of moral would pause before breaking a promise—perhaps a promise, any promise, to his wife—and ask himself whether he would wish that the maxim on which he was about to act (that it is right for husbands to break promises they make to their wives) should become a universal law. In these cases Kant was convinced that the actor would reflect on this possibility and would conclude that it is simply wrong to will that this maxim should apply universally. What would the institution of marriage be like if this were to be the case? For Kant, the stern moral philosopher, there could be no exceptions. And it is not just a case of not wishing that such a maxim be universalized, rather it is simply impossible to universalize it. Kant could not conceive how any rational person could universalize a maxim that it is right to break promises. Consequently, it followed for Kant that it is wrong in every instance to break a promise to one's wife.

What are modern health workers to make of Kant's moral philosophy? One reaction might be that Kant's work could provide a significant advance towards providing a code of practice for health workers that is not authoritarian and laid down by others for health workers to follow, but allows each health worker some responsibility to apply Kant's formulae. But this expectation is quickly dashed when one realizes the severity of Kant's advice. In the complex and surprising world of modern health care the ability to be flexible, to be able to make judgements about intensely complicated ethical problems rapidly under pressure, and to arrive at just compromises, is essential to the best health work. But Kant's imperatives, and this central doctrine, are unyielding. Just as there are occasions in which a strong argument can be made out that it is the best moral choice to break a promise to one's wife or husband (perhaps you promised that if she ever again came home after midnight without letting you know then you would throw her suitcases, her clothes, her cat, and her 127 copies of *Harper's and Queen* out of the window, and it turns out that her car has broken down in the wilds), so a strong argument can often be given for making an exception to a rule which is normally used to guide moral choosing. Usually the argument will hinge on the probability that better consequences will follow from making an exception.

So Kant's position has two related difficulties. The first is that it is so uncompromising. There can be no exceptions to the duty to keep a promise, or to tell the truth, or whatever the duty is that in the abstract any rational person must will to be a universal law. If it is right to keep a promise in one instance then it must also be right to keep a promise in any other instance. The second difficulty is that Kant's principle does not take sufficient account of the consequences of actions in context. Although Kant must have reflected that the consequences of obeying the imperatives and doing one's duty were desirable, this reflection seems to have occurred on an intellectual rather than a pragmatic level.

It is not difficult to think of exceptions to the sorts of duty that Kant imagined should be moral law. Consider the duty to act on the maxim 'tell the truth', which the rational person must will to be universal law:

Following a road accident a man has been badly injured and regains consciousness in a hospital bed. He is critically ill and fighting for his life. Most medical doctors would argue that they have a duty not to tell him the truth, that his three daughters and his wife have been killed, until his condition is no longer critical, and the news is not likely to endanger his life (a different deliberation is required if it becomes obvious that the man is to die).

Further objections

As has been seen in the earlier part of this book, the nature of ethics is indistinct. There are several alternative senses in which morality can be used, ranging from definitions to cope with the specific dramatic dilemmas, to senses of morality which inspire general and persisting questions about how people should live. Kant did not establish the difference between morality and immorality clearly enough by his various doctrines. Without a clear definition it becomes possible to offer some very spurious justifications for behaviour which most theories of ethics would not accept as moral. For instance, it is possible to will that the maxim 'No one should steal' should become a universal law. But the person who wills this might do so entirely out of self-interest. She might have a large house, a good job, and money in the bank, and be interested only in maintaining this position. Only the doctrine of 'egotism' has offered such an unusual account of morality, and it is far from clear that this is part of the realm of ethical theory at all.

Kant's main intention was to argue that people should not make deceitful promises, and then break them to suit their own ends. A classic example of such deceit occurs when a person promises to repay a loan and then absconds with the money. However, even obedience to the duty not to make deceitful promises (or not to break promises) need not be the most moral course of action in every case in practice. For example, perhaps the borrowed money has been lent by a corrupt government which presides over a society in which people are tortured. The borrowed money is then used to fund a charity campaigning against torture, and there is an associated moral advantage that the loss of the money will help disable the corrupt government. It is legitimate to agree with Kant that whatever the consequences it is morally important to abide by a pure motive to do one's duty, but such a stance is hard, if not impossible to justify in such exceptional practical instances. Being moral is surely more than simply following rules and obeying abstract duties. Attempting to be as moral as possible is difficult—it demands good intention but it also demands thought, foresight, logic, detachment, and integrity—human qualities just as precious as the faculty of pure reason.

One further problem with Kant's moral philosophy is that the *principle of ends* is incomplete and inadequate as advice on how a person can act in the most moral way. If a person attempts to adopt the principle of ends he will inevitably be faced with situations in life where he will be in contact with a number of people, all of whom have a claim to be treated as ends, yet it will not be possible to treat them all as ends. Kant's idealism again runs into problems in practice. More substantial advice is necessary, but it is not forthcoming. If, for instance, a scarce resource exists which can be permitted to only a proportion of people who could benefit from it, then the actor who is in a position to distribute this resource, and who wishes to treat all these potential recipients as ends, is in an impossible position. For instance, she may be an admissions tutor at university, and she may dearly wish to admit all who are qualified and have applied to her degree course, But, due to government cuts, these places are severely limited, and so only some of the applicants can have their wishes respected and be treated as ends. The remainder, no matter how kind the letter of rejection, are discarded as if they are of no account.

If a person fails to treat as ends all those he might have treated as ends, then he has offended against the moral law as Kant perceived it. And what is more, the principle of ends offers no criterion as a means to decide which of the people should be treated as ends if everyone cannot be.

What features should health workers note most of all about Kant's ethical theory?

The core of Kant's moral philosophy is that, once a person is in tune with his moral conscience, it is a relatively simple matter to act in the most moral way. For Kant moral issues are not complex or insoluble—ethics is not a frustrating form of cerebral perpetual motion—rather it is possible for a person to be moral, and moral in exactly the same way as all other persons within the 'moral community', by using a faculty that is possessed uniquely by human beings: namely the faculty of reason. By reflection and introspection it is possible, according to Kant, to discover laws of morality. It is possible for mature human beings without mental defects to discover certain imperatives, certain rules they must abide by if they are to be moral. Thus the emphasis is placed on human reason to reflect upon and discover what is moral. It is not enough simply to obey rules because it is legal or because it is part of your job (so those who carry out immoral instructions from their superiors can have no moral defence for their actions according to Kant). Personal motive is crucial. Thus emphasis is placed upon the responsibility of individuals to discover the pure motives (the moral path) for themselves, and sometimes in spite of external pressure to the contrary. Health workers who insist on following instructions and codes because it is expedient for them to do so may find something in Kant's work to move them to revise their opinions.

Another linchpin of Kant's moral philosophy is the idea of *universalizability*—that if a rule or law is moral in one context for one person then it must follow that the rule or law will always be moral in any context and for any persons. It is important for health workers to note that the idea of universalizability rests on the notion that all people are *equal* in crucial respects, whatever their position and circumstances in life. Consequently, it is fundamentally immoral to act towards one person or group of persons in situation X whilst acting differently towards other persons also in situation X, whatever the possible external justification. What is so impressive about Kant's work is his insistence that all people should be treated as ends acting within a community in which all other people are equal as moral agents, or potential moral agents, and entitled to equal respect because of this—whatever their economic status or whatever their age or physical condition. (There were some exceptions; for instance, criminals should be punished according to Kant because, through their crimes, he considered that they had sacrificed the right to be treated as ends. This part of his argument is opposed to the rationale of work for health presented in this book.)

So, Kant emphasizes individual responsibility and the belief that people ought to be treated as equals, since we all share the uniquely human ability to reason morally. This fact transcends all our material differences. What is less useful to health workers is Kant's theory that individual responsibility and freedom to make the best moral judgements possible stops at the point where universalizable rules are discovered. In the fraught world of health care the best decision is not always made according to some general law that has been universalized. There will be cases in which the human interest will be best served by suspending 'moral laws' (arguably, such a case occurr two world wars). And there will be cases in which choices have to be made abou persons to do good to when not everyone can be helped.

Finally, the most significant inadequacy of Kant's theory—an inadequacy that he workers cannot afford to ignore—is the underemphasis on a consideration of conse- quences. In the real world it is simply not a defence, either morally or legally, to say that what was done was done out of a pure motive to be moral. Considerations of logic, probability of outcome, and actual outcome must enter the picture when the degree of morality is assessed. A more complete view of morality comes into play when the consequences are considered. The moral realm concerns more than pure motive, just as in law where conspiracy to murder (intent to murder) and actual murder (where the consequence is that life is lost) are different crimes with different punishments. And outside the legal sphere, intent to be kind to another person is not the same thing as actually being kind to her. Actually being kind to a person shows a higher degree of morality.

The Ethic of Consequences

What is consequentialism and what is utilitarianism?

For the sake of clarity it is important to explain the difference between consequentialism and utilitarianism. Consequentialism is the more global ethical theory. Utilitarianism is a major subset of the global category. Such are the similarities between the principles of the two theories that it is sufficient to introduce consequentialism, and to direct the majority of the discussion to utilitarianism.

Consequentialism

On the face of it consequentialism is a straightforward doctrine, apparently diametri- cally opposed to the type of deontology advocated by Kant. The most radical form of consequentialism holds that the rightness or wrongness of an act should be judged only on the ground of whether its consequences produce more benefits than disadvantages. The nature of the consequences that can be thought of as either beneficial or disadvan- tageous will have been defined beforehand by the consequentialist. A consequentialist will decide how she should act by assessing the likely outcomes of her proposed action, and will judge the ultimate morality of what she has or has not done according to how her action turns out.

Utilitarianism

Utilitarianism is classically associated with the goal of happiness or pleasure. However, in the debates between moral philosophers in this century such a simple measure has come to be considered as rather crude. Other measures of utility are now considered to be legitimate, so that at times it is artificial to distinguish between utilitarianism and consequentialism.

Unlike deontological theories, utilitarianism does not depend upon duties and principles which are meant to have the authority of commandments. Utilitarianism, by contrast, is a prescription for action which does not assume that there are naturally right things to do. Utilitarianism is not concerned with motives for actions, but with the results of actions. At its simplest the utilitarian prescription for action is this: a person ought always to act in such a way that will produce the greatest balance of good over evil.

What is 'good' and what is 'evil'? The definition of these terms will vary, but will usually centre on some idea that human fulfilment is desirable and its opposite is not. The earliest form of utilitarianism defined the 'good' as 'pleasure' or 'happiness'. The 'greatest happiness principle' of Jeremy Bentham (who, along with Mill, is most usually associated with utilitarianism) states that a person should attempt to achieve 'the greatest good, or greatest happiness, of the greatest number' (although this formula does not make it clear whether or not the good should be distributed as widely and equally as possible, or is best concentrated in the hands of a few people who will benefit greatly and whose collective happiness might outweigh the collective happiness of the mass). One alternative definition of the utilitarian good was proposed by G.E. Moore who thought, presumably on the basis of his own preferences, that the central human goods were personal relationships and aesthetic experiences.

But what it is most important to note about utilitarianism is that whatever the definition of 'good' and 'evil' these 'goods' and 'evils' must be *measurable*. It is crucial to utilitarianism that a cost–benefit calculation can be made. The extent of the balance between good and evil cannot depend only upon subjective opinion, rather the calculation must be measurable according to agreed standards laid down beforehand.

Utilitarianism does not hold that the highest good is the good of the self; this would be a form of egotism. Utilitarianism insists that the agent himself must be considered as a person of equal importance with all others (and no more) in the assessment of the likely balance between good and evil. As Mill argues, 'The utilitarian standard of what is right in conduct is not the agent's own happiness but that of all considered. As between his own happiness and that of others, utilitarianism requires him to be as strictly impartial as a disinterested and benevolent spectator' (Mill 1910, p. 18). Utilitarianism requires that a person should sacrifice his self-interest if this is likely to bring about an increase in the general good. For Mill an agent's basic duty rests in the requirement to assess the consequences of actions in relation to the overall good of the species of which we are a part.

(Note: it is an error to think of deontologists and consequentialists as making up some sort of tribe, hunting in packs like dingoes, always acting precisely in accord with the dictates of the particular moral theory to which they subscribe. In reality those who write about and espouse technical ethics treat the subject like a game. For the sake of argument or prestige a person will defend a particular position to the hilt—for instance, the person might argue that in every possible circumstance his idiosyncratic version of act-utilitarianism is always the most moral option—but rarely, if ever, will this position be carried into the everyday life of the philosopher.

Following from this it is not proposed that health workers become card-carrying utilitarians or deontologists. But it is necessary that health workers are acquainted with the bones of these traditional moral theories in order that they occupy a position from which they are able to take the fullest advantage of the Ethical Grid, using it to help them deliberate over moral issues as comprehensively as possible.)

Types of utilitarianism

Act-utilitarianism

The type of utilitarianism known as act-utilitarianism states that in each situation that he is part of a person should, if he is to do the right thing, assess which of the actions open to him is most likely to produce the greatest balance of 'the good' (however defined) over 'evil'. Unlike 'acting morally' according to the ideas of deontology, moral activity for act-utilitarianism is not a case of acting according to a 'pure motive' or according to a prior duty. Rather it falls to the act-utilitarian, in each case he faces, to ask: 'What effect will my action have on the amount of good in the world?' Where a deontologist might insist that in all cases it is a moral duty to keep promises, an act-utilitarian would not take this for granted at all. Instead, in the light of the unique and specific prevailing circumstances, she will weigh up the pros and cons of keeping the promise, always giving the fullest possible attention to a consideration of the likely outcome in terms of the balance of good over evil. If the action in the particular set of circumstances does not seem likely to produce a balance of good over evil then the person is justified—according to act-utilitarianism—in breaking the promise. Act-utilitarian thinking need not be quite as crude as this since act-utilitarians also need to include in their calculation the likely effects on other people caused by the glib breaking of a promise for the sake of expedience. It may be that the decrease in general levels of integrity is not a price worth paying even in act-utilitarian terms.

The single abiding principle of act-utilitarianism is that in each case the person contemplating doing something, or nothing, should weigh up the benefits and disadvantages in terms of creating more or less of the predefined 'good'. As such act-utilitarianism can best be described as a form of opportunism. It does not accept any rules other than the requirement to calculate (although there is a modified form of act-utilitarianism which permits 'rules of thumb' based on past experiences—to avoid the absurdity of having to calculate afresh on each occasion). If, on balance, the likely outcome of your intended action is a balance of good over evil, then do it! Do it whatever it is, even if it is stealing, or lying, or harming somebody physically, or destroying some people emotionally, or blackmailing, or breaking the law of the land, or murdering someone, or betraying a friend—or taking a two-week package holiday in Benidorm. If the action will produce more good than evil in the end, then that is what you should do.

What are the relevant issues for health workers of act-utilitarianism? First, it is difficult to imagine any national system of medicine and health care advocating that its staff adopt the philosophy of act-utilitarianism. For instance, 'health workers' who applied the theory with enthusiasm might seek to justify a lower standard of care—or involuntary euthanasia for old people occupying beds that could be used to treat younger people in need of care. Such discrimination, although possibly justifiable in utilitarian terms, is alien to the rationale of work for health and also might well lead to litigation.

There is a further practical problem. The act-utilitarian must assess, in each and every case, the likely ratio of good and evil. Yet it seems that this requirement is simply unrealistic in the urgent and complicated world of health work. What is needed is a way of reflection that does not demand calculation afresh in every case, yet which still retains a major element of individual responsibility.

And it is this focus on individual responsibility to assess actions and outcomes of actions that is the main benefit of act-utilitarianism. Just as act-deontology places emphasis on a person having a basic duty to herself, a duty to judge and to reflect on the whole array of principles and possibilities available, so act-utilitarianism can act as a compelling reminder to a health worker that the rules of practice which she has learnt, or the rules that are handed out to her by her superior, are not necessarily rules that ought to be obeyed in all cases. The given rules might be disobeyed if the health worker calculates that to obey them in a specific case will produce a balance of evil over good (or at least a less beneficial balance than might otherwise be obtained). In some cases (perhaps the house rule is never to explain to patients what their treatment is) sticking to the rules might produce consequences that are considered to be an unacceptable price to pay for the sake of doing one's duty and being consistent.

General utilitarianism

This version of utilitarianism talks neither about unique responses to specific situations, nor about rules. General utilitarianism asks that any potential actor should ask himself, 'What if everyone were to do what I propose to do?' For example, a doctor of medicine who is about to deceive a patient about his condition should ask himself what the consequences would be if everyone deceived one another about information they believe the other person would not like to hear.

General utilitarianism is not a particularly complicated doctrine. Most people have said to someone about to do something of which they disapprove, 'What if everybody did that?' and there is real worth in this dictum of common sense. However, in the context of health work the theory is a little incomplete. It should be used as a stimulus to thought. For instance, recall the case of Diane, the Health Visitor (Chapter Four), whose rationale for her work was not that she produce the highest possible proportion of child immunizations, but rather that she helped as many people as possible to think through their situations to enable them to weigh up the pros and cons of vaccinating their children. For Diane the highest priority was not a possible decrease in disease and illness, but a possible increase in the level of education of the people with whom she worked. The problem is that the response to Diane's work practice 'But what if everyone did that?' is commonplace amongst community nurses. The argument is that if all health visitors saw their role as remedial educators rather than medical workers then this might have bad consequences for the health service whose level of future funding depends in part upon the sort of 'performance indicator' that good immunization rates produce. And how would general practitioners react to an army of rebel 'nurse educators'?

However, the response 'What if everybody did that?' is not damning. It is equally up to those nurses who think of their work in the sort of terms that Diane conceives the profession to ask those who view immunization work as a 'sales campaign' 'What if everybody did that?' General utilitarianism has most importance as an impetus to personal reflection. It is an aid to debate which places strong emphasis on the consequences of actions.

Rule-utilitarianism

In a manner which resembles the advice given by rule-deontology, rule-utilitarianism argues that it is not personal judgement but obedience to certain rules that is fundamental to morality. But where most forms of rule-deontology insist that the rules exist *a priori* (that is, rules of conduct exist prior to human experience), rule-utilitarianism asserts that rules of conduct are to be discovered through a process of calculation in order to discover which rules, if always adhered to, will produce the greatest balance of good over evil. This process is not carried out in the abstract. For this version of utilitarianism the justification for rules is to be found in their utility rather than their purity. This proviso apart, there are marked similarities of application between rule-deontology and rule-utilitarianism.

In contrast to act-utilitarianism, where it can be acceptable to maintain rules—but only as a general guideline—rule-utilitarianism stresses that always to keep a certain rule will be to produce the greatest good in the long run. So, the rule-utilitarian will calculate that the best consequences will result, for example, from obedience to the rule always to tell the truth. The difference between act-utilitarianism and rule-utilitarianism can be indicated in this way:

A health education officer friend (you too are a health education officer) has stolen items from the stationery store regularly over the last two years, and you have been aware of this. Most people you know have done something like this in the past, and it is not regarded by most people as a serious crime. It is seen more as a perk of the job. However, your District Medical Officer asks you a direct question, namely: 'Has Alberto stolen the coloured duplicating paper that was meant for those urgent posters on healthy bowels?' You know that he has and you know also that if you tell the truth your friend's job will be in danger.

It is likely, although not certain, that an act-utilitarian would say that in this case utility demands that a lie be told in the interest of Alberto and his family—after all it is only a minor misdemeanour—while a rule-utilitarian would insist that the truth be told on the ground that it is better that the truth is always told than that it is broken, even though there might be more benefit in this case in the short term from telling a lie.

What are the relevant issues for health workers of rule-utilitarianism?   The major benefit that might be derived from health workers following the theory of rule-utilitarianism is that they will be working under rules arrived at through a careful consideration of the consequences of actions, based on a thorough review of past costs and benefits.

The central problem that health workers have to face if they choose this single theory of ethics is a difficulty which plagues all varieties of utilitarianism. It is this. There may well be occasions in which the rule of utility creates an excess of good over evil for a population taken as a whole, but does not distribute this good fairly. It may be that although more good than evil is produced in general, a certain proportion of a population might actually suffer rather than gain, but their suffering will be outweighed by the gains made by other members of the population. Thus a principle of justice (that it is right that all goods should be distributed equally) is undermined by utilitarianism. For example, many members of the British Labour Party argue that such a calculation has been made by the Tory Government of the 1980s. The argument is that the governmment sees great utilitarian advantage in maintaining a high level of unemployment (the unions are kept under control because there is an endemic fear of unemployment, output increases, and there is an increasing standard of living for those in employment)—the majority enjoy benefit whilst the minority suffer, and on utilitarian terms this is right.

To take a health service example, it might serve utility to relocate from hospitals all non-dangerous sufferers from mental illness within the community (it might save money, it might make many patients happier and better adjusted), but if such a policy is carried out consistently and without room for exceptions within the qualifying category (to make only a few exceptions could prove disproportionately expensive) then inevitably there will be a number of patients, relatives, and carers who suffer.

The classic illustration of how utilitarianism can appear unpalatable to those who hold *justice as fairness* as a fundamental ethical principle has been given in this form:

> ... let us imagine that the happiness of the whole human race were to be immeasurably increased—poverty eliminated, brotherhood achieved, disease conquered ... but the condition is that one man, his life mysteriously prolonged, is to be kept involuntarily in a state of continuous and agonising torture. According to the utilitarian criterion, which measures the rightness of an act by its results, it would seem that the argument is justified ... the net balance of the utilitarian moral scale would have to point in the direction of maximum happiness and away from the eternal agony of the single suffering man. But most people who consider the proposed bargain feel that there is something terribly wrong with it. (Raphael 1981)

There is a further significant problem with utilitarianism in general. It arises because, logically, utilitarians must claim that any action is right so long as it brings about favourable consequences—even if the intention of the actor was clearly evil and immoral. For instance, imagine that a medical doctor practising cosmetic surgery privately had, through deliberate cost-cutting, disfigured nearly 50 patients, two of whom were driven to suicide because of the results of the surgeon's poor technique. This malpractice comes to light and as a result the doctor is struck off the medical register, compensation is paid to all the victims, and most important of all, a thorough policing operation of all advertisers of cosmetic surgery is carried out in future. This ensures that this form of malpractice can never occur again, thus sparing potentially thousands of people unnecessary suffering. Since this is the outcome, in utilitarian terms the actions of the corrupt doctor have to be defined as 'moral' despite the immoral intent. Such incongruity is hard to reconcile unless utilitarians are prepared to dilute their theories with aspects of other moral theories. But if this is done then this approach can no longer be described as utilitarian.

Justice

In addition to the basic grounding in ethical theory contained in Chapters Three and Four it is necessary to provide an outline of a principle that is often used in moral debate about health work: the *principle of justice*.

What is justice?   This is a question which is at least as difficult to provide an answer to as the question 'What is health?' What is certain is that it is not possible to give a definitive answer. Just as with 'health' there are a number of legitimate uses of the word 'justice', all of which might stake a claim to be 'the true meaning', but none of which can or should ever finally become primary since it is only in multiplicity that the richest sense of justice can be comprehended.

Commonly, justice is thought of in two ways: justice as 'fairness' and justice as 'appropriate punishment for wrongdoing'. Justice as fairness is usually thought to have been offended against if, for instance, in a relationship which is supposed to be a partnership (a marriage, for example) one of the partners is manifestly getting more of the benefits even though she has not contributed more than the other partner. Justice as appropriate punishment for wrongdoing is described, in the technical language of some philosophers, as 'retributive justice'—the justice of retribution for perceived offence. This second aspect of justice is not of concern for this inquiry.

Three versions of 'justice as fairness'

There are three interesting ways of subdividing the idea of justice as fairness. All have a legitimate claim to be included as an aspect of the overall notion of justice, but only one (with its implication of respect and equality) is *fundamental* to a true health service. The three types are (in all cases the justice referred to is justice thought of in relation to individuals): 'to each according to his rights', 'to each according to what he deserves', and 'to each according to his need'. Of these it is the final dictum that represents the idea of justice that should be associated with the richest sense of work for health (see Miller 1976 for a full analysis of this topic).

The idea of justice which lies behind the expression 'to each according to his rights' is the idea of contract. For example, if a person agrees to labour for a particular sum of money it is his right, and it is just, that his employer actually pays him his due (so long as the worker has abided by the specific conditions of the contract: he has, for instance, got to have done the job properly as agreed).

The idea of justice which informs the expression 'to each according to what he deserves' is that which is used to justify meritocracies, where the people who have worked the hardest or most successfully are rewarded with the most benefits, in proportion to their efforts and their merit. If a person puts in long and torturous hours building up her business then, if there is justice in this sense, she deserves to reap the harvest for her endeavours. So it is just that she eventually receives the financial rewards to which she is entitled through the merit of her labours. Similarly, if a person strives diligently to obtain good university degrees, earning little money during that time and possibly sacrificing the opportunity to earn more outside university, then—according to the idea of justice as 'to each according to his desert'—it is just that eventually he is accorded the status and earning power that all his studying and application merit.

Both the above ideas of justice are highly contentious: for instance, it is a fact in British law that people have equal rights to own property, but all people do not have property and vast inequalities of possession of property exist within most societies. This inequality persists to such an extent that it might be argued that a more basic principle of justice (perhaps that of equitable distribution of a society's resources) should override the principle of 'to each according to his right', at least in exceptional cases of inequality. Likewise with the notion of justice as 'to each according to his desert'. The claim of this principle to be basic to the idea of justice is called into question by such examples as this: perhaps the young man who has worked hard and done well at university does deserve, in one sense, to enjoy the benefits of his dedication. But this desert is at least tempered by the knowledge that he has been exceptionally privileged to have been able to attend university in the first place. Places at universities have become increasingly scarce (at least in the Britain governed by the Tory Party), and many young people have great initial advantages in the fight to obtain places. Because of factors of upbringing and environment—which bring such benefits as earlier access to books, a wider range of parental vocabulary, and different peer pressures—middle-class children have a far higher chance of attending university than their working-class contemporaries, even though their basic talents might be equivalent. The existence of such inequalities as this can significantly undermine the claims to be fundamental of the options of justice as 'to each according to his right' and 'to each according to his desert'.

The above discussion is painfully superficial, and it is also arguable that the idea of justice as 'to each according to his need' has inadequacies which are at least as serious. However, it is part of the argument of this book that it should be one of four basic principles of a health service. Indeed this principle, and not the alternative options under 'justice as fairness', is already espoused as basic by many people who are working for health. Many contemporary health workers do what they do because they wish to do justice: not primarily in the sense of ensuring that contracts are honoured (although this factor is clearly important in various ways), and certainly not in the sense that treatment and care is given only to those who are considered to deserve it or to have earned it on merit, or that better care is given to those who deserve it most of all; but instead many health workers are driven by the desire to help people—any person, whoever he is or whatever he has done with his life—overcome physical and mental problems when they are not able to do so unaided. True work for health concentrates first and foremost on people's needs (within certain limits: see Seedhouse 1986, pp. 64–8)—whether these are food or warmth or shelter or surgery or kindness or advice or education or love—and it is informed by a notion of justice which regards the fulfilment of need, equally and without discrimination, as a fundamental premise of work for health (see the Ethical Grid).

A developed notion of justice—Rawls and 'justice as fairness'

Although the principle of justice cannot be given a full analysis in this book, it is such a central notion in health work that it is important to introduce the work of an influential modern philosopher in this area—John Rawls. Rawls worked out an elaborate system which he thought might work to ensure a just social organizaton (Rawls 1973).

The just society arising from a veil of ignorance   Rawls's theory is complicated, and by no means all its details are relevant to the set task of this inquiry. Fundamentally Rawls insists that central to the proper sense of justice is the idea that the existence of unequal possession and distribution of such desired qualities as power, wealth, and income are simply impermissible in a society unless these inequalities actually work to the absolute benefit of the worst-off members of a society.

As the means of demonstrating the strength of this claim Rawls asks us to imagine ourselves in a hypothetical situation. This is that each of us is a free, logical, yet disinterested being about to enter into a *social contract* with everyone else in order to form a just society. The fascinating feature about Rawls's proposal is that none of the parties to the contract knows what or where they will be in the society. The social contract is to be made behind a veil of ignorance. This veil conceals completely the place of each individual in the society—no one knows what their place or condition will be. They might be male or female, young or old, employer or employee, rich man or poor man, diseased or not.

After asking us to imagine this veil of ignorance Rawls throws down a challenge to the potential social contractors behind the veil of ignorance: which principles should the society espouse in order to be just?

It is well worth reflecting personally about this challenge. All moral questions are implicit within the structure and organization of any society.

Briefly, Rawls's own answer to the challenge is this:

There are to be two main principles of justice in the society. The first of these is to take priority over the second if there are any instances of conflict over these principles.

1. Each person is to have an equal right to the maximum amount of liberty consistent with a similar liberty for others. In other words, each person is to have the same right as anyone else to as much freedom as possible unless this freedom works against the freedoms of other people. The basic liberties according to Rawls are political liberty, the right to property, freedom from arbitrary arrest, and to be within a system of law which deals impartially with all who come under its rule.

2. Any social and economic inequalities that exist are to be arranged so that these inequalities will work to everyone's advantage, including the worst-off. The idea behind this principle is that in a modern and complex society, which is bound to contain people of different abilities, there will inevitably be some inequalities. But if these inequalities work only for the benefit of those who are already privileged then they should not be allowed. An example of a justifiable inequality, according to Rawls, is that it is permissible for a surgeon to be well-off, but only because his skills have the potential to contribute to the well-being of all, so that a society without the services of the rich surgeon will be worse off.

Rawls's argument is open to criticism. For example, it has been argued that Rawls's response to the challenge he has set up is not the only feasible conclusion that might be reached from behind the veil of ignorance. Why, for instance, does Rawls select the principle of liberty above that of equality? There is no reason to think that some social contractors behind the veil of ignorance would not conclude that the best way of ensuring justice within a society is to guarantee equal distribution of resources, even at the cost of a lower level of personal liberty in the populace. Rawls's own judgement does not appear to have been made in total ignorance, but rather has been informed by his adherence to liberal principles. Rawls makes an assumption that the 'rational person' judging from behind the veil of ignorance is actually 'rational' in a manner that is in line with broad liberal political philosophy. Independently of the question of who actually is the surgeon and who is the dustman, the ignorant 'rationalist' is supposed to think it right *a priori* that the grossly unequal roles and status of dustman and surgeon should exist in a just society. Different social structures and arrangements from those which presently make up Western society are not expected to be considered by the ignorant 'rationalist'. For example, Rawls does not envisage any person behind the veil of ignorance being prepared to argue for absolute equality of education for fear that he might then be at risk through the absence of trained surgeons. But it is by no means absurd to think that some social contractors might be prepared to bargain for a system of education that did not stream and create elite specialisms. It is possible that a different system of education might eliminate the need for so many surgeons, and it is hard to show that a more equal system of education, and more equal later financial reward, would result in a scarcity of trained surgeons.

The pros and cons of Rawls's theory of justice are not a major concern for this inquiry. But what is central to the development of the argument of this book is the powerful connection, highlighted by Rawls, that persists between politics and morality. The political and social structure of a society is profoundly and intimately linked to the level of morality that exists for the people. If the social structures are such that 'justice as fairness' can not be achieved to its fullest extent for all the people—if these social structures enable some people to achieve worthwhile potentials but do not allow other people equivalent opportunities—then morality is not being created to as full a degree a possible. It is argued in the concluding chapters of this book—where many threads of the tapestry of the account are sewn together—that since work for health is a moral endeavour, and since the rationale of health rests on a basic principle of justice, then the entire structure of the health service—its organizations, its administration, its hierarchies, its priorities, its resourcing—is of moral concern because it is directly responsible for creating or diminishing the degree of morality achieved.

Summary

Chapter Seven has given a basic account of the two classic approaches to moral reasoning: deontology and consequentialism. This, together with the more abstract discussion concerning the foundation of morality given in Chapter Five, provides health workers with sufficient background and working material to begin to reflect with confidence about moral issues, and to confront dilemmas and make interventions in a way which is both more effective and more moral. The information given in this chapter is essential if the operation and value of the Ethical Grid is to be properly understood.

Part III

'How dare you dwarf us?'

Chapter Eight
Obstacles to Clear Moral Reasoning

It is important to recognize that moral reasoning is not a simple matter, and that certain ways of thinking and calculating actually debilitate the process. In this chapter related obstacles to clear moral reasoning are discussed. In particular these are 'bad faith' and inappropriate cost–benefit analysis. The content of this chapter forms a part of the introduction to the Ethical Grid.

In order to use the Ethical Grid properly honesty is essential. True moral reasoning requires openness about one's personal motives. Personal integrity provides a natural limit to the use of the grid. The importance of integrity can be shown by concentrating on the notion of 'bad faith'. 'Bad faith' abrogates personal responsibility. 'Bad faith' is the antithesis of personal authenticity. If a person has 'bad faith' then that person can be moral only to a limited degree, at best. If a person has 'bad faith' then he denies himself, he is inauthentic, he has no integrity—yet integrity is essential to a proper use of the grid. It is essential to moral reasoning.

Bad Faith

The notion of 'bad faith' was announced by Jean-Paul Sartre. When people are guilty of 'bad faith' they are guilty of not being true to themselves, they have committed the dreadful crime of denying their individuality and unique personal freedom by burying this in a role that they play. Unfortunately, playing given roles and fitting into predefined categories are characteristics that are sometimes displayed by people who become professionals. On occasions people who take on jobs where they are defined as 'professionals' (where they have specialist skills and knowledge) change radically from how they were before. The professional's very identity—the way in which she conceives of herself—changes to fit the position she has taken on. People can become addicted to the role and idea of being a 'professional'—so much so that they think of 'professional moral responsibility' as being different from 'personal moral responsibility'. They suffer from an unfortunate but none the less socially acceptable form of schizophrenia.

Sartre said that all of us to differing degrees cope with an 'irrational world'. By the term 'irrational' Sartre means that, despite the superficial appearance of order and structure, our world is not ordered. It is random. Things happen and there is no real control over these things (rather like Nottingham Forest's defence strategy). Nothing is determined. Events are free and conform to no pattern, no logic. Our world is 'irrational' since our canons of rationality, logic, order, and coherence are appearance only and not real at all. Reality is actually chaotic, meaningless, and without order. We categorize the world. We categorize ourselves. If we did not we would feel permanently disorientated—dizzy—we would be anguished and nauseous, but at least we would retain our full capacity for free choice. We would at least retain our true selves.

Bad faith is essentially the denial of our freedom of choice, and as such it is the denial of our ability to make moral judgements. If we see ourselves as bound to act in a certain way, if we feel inclined to say, 'I have no choice in this matter', then we are deceiving ourselves. Bad faith is a self-deception which makes us believe that acting out a role is really being authentic. It is a self-deceit that creates the belief that all our behaviour is determined by the role we play. Bad faith is the failure to realize that even the role we play has originally been a matter of choice, and that it remains a matter of choice whether to continue in the role or not.

There are degrees of bad faith. It may be exhibited when a person buys a luxury item—perhaps a watch with a plain granite face—and justifies the purchase by saying that it was essential, or when a person does nothing politically, claiming that she was brought up to be apolitical. And there are many people (perhaps all of us) who always see themselves as a particular stereotype—as the dutiful housewife with two children, cooking meals at set times for her husband, just as her mother did before her; or as the kindly paternalistic general practitioner; or as the angry, certain, righteous member of Militant; or as the total feminist; or as the idle erudite philosopher sponging a good wage from the State, always 'writing a book' but never finishing it. The point is that all their tastes, beliefs, and actions are dictated not by themselves but by the role that they are playing.

Sartre thought that the man who exhibits bad faith does so in order to stop being a person, in order to become an object instead. In this way creativity is totally sacrificed for the sake of the security of a tried and trusted role. The man who has bad faith tries to become an object in order to lose true consciousness. As a result he abdicates responsibility. He throws away choice for the sake of becoming a pawn, determined to operate only in predetermined predictable ways. Bad faith is a personal disgrace.

Crucially if there is no real choice then there can be no moral development. Moral development depends upon integrity which cannot exist at the same time as bad faith. The point that Sartre can be seen to be emphasizing is that no matter what the rules or how tight the bureaucracy and professional role, or selected personal role, there is always choice. Not to believe this is to atrophy and ossify into an object—which is the worst crime that a person can ever commit against himself.

Although much of Sartre's philosophy is difficult to accept—and it certainly is not being argued here that health professionals should really view the world as irrational and chaotic—his insight into bad faith is illuminating. It has powerful ramifications for the ways in which it is possible for individuals to act morally within large and complex organizations.

Essence and existence—an expansion

The central concern of this book is the question: What are human beings for? What is it about human beings that makes our existence truly worthwhile, and what degrades us? This is not a question that can be finally proved or refuted 'scientifically', but it is one that can be discussed so that meaningful conclusions can be reached.

Sartre's contribution is important for this analysis in two ways. First, Sartre has asserted the existence of a unique capacity in people—the capacity for free and autonomous choice. And further, the existence of this capacity has major implications for the way in which societies, and their internal institutions, are organized and structured. The crucial question is: To what extent does a society and its institutions enable this capacity, effectively, in the human beings who compose it?

Another way of posing this question is to ask: To what extent does a society permit its members to overcome the tendency to bad faith? To what extent are those with power in a society happy for the majority of people to be 'objects' in Sartre's terms? How many people can be permitted to exist freely?

Sartre made a fundamental distinction between people and objects. Objects, for instance chairs or satchels, have an essence—what they are is predetermined. Their nature is fixed according to their given function. However, people are not and should not be like this. They do not have a predetermined essence—a given function—a 'shape' like an object. All people have is existence. This fact allows an unadulterated freedom for a person to create herself—not according to a set pattern, but uniquely. This is a frightening freedom that many people do not feel able to face up to, preferring instead to believe that they are essences.

Clearly this case is simplistic. For instance, it takes no account of genetic potentials, neither does it recognize that people do not have infinite potential, and nor does it appreciate that people can be greatly constrained by external circumstances and events (as Sartre was to realize later in his life). Rather it is the moral principle that Sartre has highlighted that is important.

A further problem

It is a fact of life that many people, often it seems to be the overwhelming majority, are content to be instructed. Not everyone wants to take responsibility, not everyone is inclined to take risks and to be creative. Some people insist that there is much that they would rather not know, even about medical treatments that are done to them. Many people are trusting and submissive and are happy to have their horizons defined for them. Some people do not want autonomy because it is taxing, and it can hurt. Why should not people spend their lives in cotton wool if that is what they wish? Why should not people decide autonomously to abdicate their autonomy in favour of being looked after by the State, an institution, or another person?

There are two reasons, one of them practical, why the talent of personal deliberation and independent choosing should be encouraged in all forms of human life, including professional life. A person who has been trained habitually to follow given rules will be badly underdeveloped as a person. An essential part of her will be left barren when it could be verdant and flourishing. She will not be able to choose for herself on her own terms. If the indoctrination has been overdone then there will be a problem about making any choices. Even when a person operates under a system of rules there is still a need for a degree of choice and deliberation. Is this a situation of the kind in which I should apply this rule? In this case, is this procedure justified? Which of the rules that I could use should I choose?

The practical reason why bad faith should be extinguished is that such a human being is not properly equipped to deal with the unexpected and unique situations in life. And these are the sorts of situations that face health workers. The unique case, the surprising and novel issue (perhaps an issue raised by advances in medical technology), the urgent problem when there is no time to consult the rule book or to refer to a superior—all these things will occur from time to time. It is in these instances that only the person who has been able to develop his sense of judgement can act at all—committed rule-followers must stand by helplessly, redundant without their guide. Those who have the conviction to think for themselves are in a far better position. They can follow rules if they believe that it is wise to do so, but they have the great advantage of being able to override these rules—taking autonomous responsibility—if they believe that this is what should be done. And it is not so difficult to imagine what it could be like to throw off the shackles of bad faith.

An illustration   There is an enlightening illustration of the dizziness, the sense of being a stranger in a foreign land, the freedom and the fear, that people can experience when they first try to shake off their bad faith. Yet the illustration is so mundane, and the step so small.

When driving road vehicles it is the law that we must stop at traffic signals on the signal red. For the good reasons of avoiding accidents and ensuring that the traffic flows smoothly it can be important to obey this particular rule. However, occasionally the traffic lights fail and we have to make our own judgement about whether or not it is safe to proceed. So it is for the best that we can choose to disobey signals that are stuck if we need to.

But this is not the most interesting case. Sometimes we are not sure if the traffic lights are working properly. Perhaps it is late at night, there is little traffic, and the lights seem to have been on red for a very long time. The rule-follower's car is four cars away from the front of the queue. Then, hesitantly, the leading car begins to move forward despite the red light. It moves away and, again hesitantly, the next car follows, and then the third car. What is the committed rule-follower to do?

Once he decides to move it will be like a revelation. Almost magically the rules will melt away, the silly red traffic light will become metal and glass and electrics. The rules will be seen as temporary, man-made, expedient, and of minor importance. The rule is not necessary at all, even though it is usually useful. It can be superseded by human judgement. The rule-follower will have been given a glimpse of what it feels like to begin to lose bad faith.

An objection

It might well be argued that this attention to the idea of bad faith is fanciful and unrealistic. One has only to observe how many people in a society accept so many of its rules without question. Many people do not even understand that questions are possible. For instance, in Britain most people accept that the British version of democracy is the only true democracy, that education for most children should cease at the age of sixteen, and countless other traditions. Since it seems to most people that these traditions have always been a part of British life there seems to be simply no other way.

A response

However, a strong case can be made out that just as the belief that things in Britain have always been more or less as they are now is mythical, so it is a myth that most people can deal only with rules. Anyone who employs moral reasoning properly—weighing and balancing rules, principles, and consequences against each other in order to obtain the best possible outcome—transcends what has been given to them. And since most health professionals perform this intellectual operation frequently it is likely that most of the general population is similarly equipped to use personal judgement, standing back from the rules.

And it is also not accurate to say that most people cannot on occasions recognize the absurdity and the transient nature of the world. Not everyone is an existentialist of Sartre's calibre (happily) but people do become aware of the fragility of existence, and the impermanence of even the aspects of life that they hold most dear. Because of this it is both right and practical to say to people: 'Here is a tool—it is not something which can give you answers that are certain because, as with so much in life, nothing is certain in the moral realm. It is up to you to use your own judgement.'

None of this is provable. The assertion is clearly open to question. If the assertion is wrong then it is probably a waste of time to provide a general tool to enhance ethical deliberation. But it is at least plausible that the ability to see beyond convention and apparent order is not a talent that is possessed by some people and not others—as some people are able to use mathematics and other people are not—but is an essential part of human intellectual make-up. All people, unless they die at an early age, can become aware that familiar 'certainties' can be displaced. This displacement can happen, for example, when a person is suddenly made redundant after long service in a job, when parents divorce, or when someone who is close dies or leaves. Such crises force the recognition that the existence we have come to feel safe with is actually acutely brittle. People who are unable to recognize the presence of this uncertainty at *any* time are unusual. For instance, if a parent suffers the death of a child at Christmas then the trimmings, and *bonhomie*, and the tinsel will apear alien, superficial, and unreal. If they do not—if only temporarily—then this would *at least* be cause for concern for a health worker who wished to facilitate the grieving process, and may well be indicative of a severe psychological disorder.

A Further Obstacle to Clear Moral Reasoning: the Wrong Kind of Cost–Benefit Analysis—the Case of QALYS

It is easier to measure those things that can be measured most easily. But it is not always true that those things that are the most measurable are the most valuable.

> *It is the mark of the educated man and a proof of his culture that in every subject he looks for only so much precision as nature permits.*

(Aristotle 1976, p. 28).

Can QALYS be a tool for a health service?

QALYS is an acronym for Quality Adjusted Life Years. The QALY is a measure intended to produce the efficient calculation of health service priorities.

QALYS are currently controversial. The controversy can be confusing because the debate over the merits and demerits of QALYS generates very different sorts of question. It is possible to expect, and fear, different things from QALYS. Health economists, administrators with fixed budgets, doctors facing torturous choices, and moral philosophers reflecting at a safe distance concentrate on different aspects. For instance, the concern might be whether or not the QALY can be a reliable measure of the quality of a person's life; or whether QALYS can offer guidelines—or even rules—to help in efficient decision-making; or whether all that QALYS can be used for is to make implicit priorities more explicit; or whether the use of QALYS actually helps patients; or whether QALYS can be used in ways that are immoral.

What is a QALY?

In the words of Alan Williams, a founder of the QALY idea:

> The essence of a QALY is that it takes a year of healthy life expectancy to be worth 1, but regards a year of unhealthy life expectancy as worth less than 1. Its precise value is lower the worse the quality of life of the unhealthy person (which is what the 'quality adjusted' bit is all about). If being dead is worth zero, it is, in principle, possible for a QALY to be negative, i.e. for the quality of a person's life to be judged worse than being dead.
>
> The general idea is that a beneficial health care activity is one that generates a positive amount of QALYS, and that an efficient health care activity is one where the cost per QALY is as low as it can be. A high priority health care activity is one where the cost-per-QALY is low, and a low priority activity is one where the cost-per-QALY is high. (Williams 1985)

So a QALY is designed as a means of assessing the differences in the quality of life between individuals. Williams's measure assumes that a healthy life is simply one in which, in physical terms, there is a good life expectancy, no pain, and no disability. According to Williams and his colleagues, a person should be thought of as becoming less healthy if her life expectancy is reduced and her degree of disability is increased. This definition of a 'healthy life' is very crude—it looks only at a few simple features of people. It certainly might be challenged by a life prisoner, or a long-term unemployed person, who has physical fitness but little else. However, this definition of health is accepted by these people without further analysis.

In addition, the advocates of QALYS commit a logical error. They fail to notice the important distinction between the 'quality' of life and the 'value' of life. They assume that if a person's quality of life—according to this crude definition of health—decreases then it follows that the *value* of that person's life must decrease proportionately. The mistake can be illustrated by the following *non sequitur*:

1. More 'health output' (more QALYS) is achieved by spending the same amount of money on Fred as on John.
2. Better cost-effectiveness is obtained by treating Fred rather than John.
3. Therefore Fred's life has more value than John's.

The fallacy becomes clear when it is appreciated that the value of a person's life is not the same as that person's worth. This distinction rests on the distinction noted earlier between basic 'persons' and 'full persons', and owes much to John Harris' analysis. Although 'full persons'—usually flourishing human beings—can have myriad talents and differences between what they are capable of, all 'persons' have basic capacities which imply a fundamental equality. It follows that there can be no differences between the value of different people's lives seen in this light. One may be fifteen or ninety, but one's existence as a person is equally valuable. However, the QALY measure assumes that the value of human life is not fixed in this way but is a 'variable' that can change according to a person's age, ability, and social status, for instance.

What are QALYS intended to be used for?

QALYS are intended to be used for different purposes. If the measure can be made reliable then they might be used to decide which of a range of possible treatments open to a patient will bring about the most favourable 'quality of life'. Alternatively, the measure might be used to discriminate between patients in competition for a scarce resource. There are other uses lying between these extremes. What is clear is that each potential use of QALYS has to be considered individually, on its own terms. Some uses of the measure might be beneficial to health and also morally desirable, while other potential uses are clearly immoral and as such cannot count as genuine health care.

QALYS can be used in the following ways:

1. In the abstract, to clarify costs of treatment, but without generating any changes in practice.
2. To make implicit priorities explicit, so as to make thinking more self-conscious and rigorous.
3. To compare and assess treatments which could produce short-term benefit against those which could produce benefit in the long term.
4. To ensure the most cost-effective use of health service funds. For example, hip-replacement operations are said to be more cost-effective in QALY terminology than heart transplants. In *The Economist* (10 January 1987) it was noted that studies at York University had come to the conclusion that heart transplants cost over £5000 per QALY compared with £1000 for coronary by-passes and £750 for hip replacements. Since health service funding is finite it was concluded that it must be better to channel available funds into hip-replacement operations.
5. To ensure the most beneficial distribution, according to the economic rationale of QALYS, of any available scarce resource. For example, renal dialysis or a drug in short supply.
6. To select for treatment those people who might be expected to produce the most QALYS. Such selection is strongly reminiscent of the policy used by armies which treat first of all those soldiers who are likely to return to the battle the most quickly. Such a policy maximizes the benefit of the treatment funded by the army.
7. To make apparently reflective judgements simply a matter of calculation.

Against QALYS

Before considering objections to the use of QALYS it is important to place the current controversy in perspective.

The QALY debate actually represents nothing more than the swing of a pendulum between deontology and consequentialism. At present there is a stronger emphasis on the assessment of the consequences of human actions as a gauge to their worth above all else. It is to be hoped that anyone reflecting on the issues will come to appreciate the *need for a balance* between the two extremes. It is the lack of balance that makes QALYS inappropriate as a tool for moral reflection.

Jeremy Bentham invented *The Felicific Calculus*. This was a method intended to help people decide which actions to take, based on an assessment of the likely consequences. Roughly, the more pleasure the action was likely to produce the more reason to do that rather than anything else. Bentham took into account the type of pleasure, the intensity of pleasure, and the duration of pleasure, and argued for a standard scale by which to calculate. His hope was that everyone would agree on this standard. But, as is the case with QALYS, such a device was doomed to intellectual failure simply because different people have different ideas about how to rate pleasures. For example, imagine how difficult it would be for any group of people drawn from a range of backgrounds to agree about how to compare objectively the amounts of pleasure generated by reading a good novel, eating a bar of chocolate, getting drunk with friends on a Saturday night, robbing a bank, or whatever the pleasure is said to be.

In support of The Felicific Calculus it should be said that Bentham took into account the pleasures of other people, and argued that the worth of human actions should be seen in the context of how much pleasure was generated for all in a society. However, in addition to the difficulty over settling on objective measures, both the 'Calculus' and QALYS flounder in application because they can act to legitimize discrimination between people. So long as the overall balance of actions is more 'good' than 'bad' (for Bentham the 'good' is pleasure and the 'bad' pain, while for the advocates of QALYS the 'good' is more cost-effective life and the 'bad' expensive life) then the actions are said to be justified.

Both ways of calculation can offend deeply against the principle of 'justice as fairness'. It is worth recalling an illustration to emphasize the point. The illustration challenges any philosophy of action which looks only at consequences and particular favoured outcomes. If we were given the choice of having a disease-free, war-free, content, and productive society at the single cost of knowing that one human being, who would be kept alive for ever, would suffer eternal and perpetual agony of mind and body, what should we choose? Consequentialists and some economists have little hesitation in agreeing to the contract—indeed their hands are forced by the requirement to be consistent—yet others tend to recoil at the injustice of such a situation. The principle of justice as fairness is revealed as a strong impulse in human life when the choice is cast this starkly, yet the QALY measure makes no room for it.

The following specific points can be made against QALYS:

1. The selection of the measure is arbitrary   The selection of the criteria of which QALYS are composed—degree of pain, length of expected life, and degree of disability—is at worst totally arbitrary, and at best governed by a 'health service' pre-occupied with economics, mortality, and morbidity. There is no objective reason why these criteria should have been chosen before, for example, intelligence, amount of past income, amount of body hair, height, or eye colour. Why not these measures? If a person was unfortunate enough to be completely bald, quite small, rather stupid, and to have been unemployed for a long time we might conclude that her quality of life is low, and so treat someone else with whatever scarce resource we have.

But this selection of criteria would quickly be condemned as an unfair and arbitrary discrimination, with the discrimination operating solely according to a person's bad luck to be as she is. But this is precisely what the QALY measure does. The criteria might sound more objective, gaining credibility from the medical context, but they have been selected, for reasons of economy rather than human equality, from an indefinite range of alternatives. If you are old or disabled or in pain or immobile—tough luck. It does not matter that you devote your life to charity—you are 78 and you are simply not worth as much as the 25 year old yuppie business man with two children.

2. Subjective values are intended to be imposed upon other people   It is possible that the use of QALYS to discriminate between people will mean that this arbitrary or biased selection of criteria will be imposed on people who might wish to live, might wish to receive the available treatment, and might well measure their own quality of life in a different way from those who assume to impose QALYS.

3. QALYS promote a myth   The myth is this:

(a) That it is possible to be certain about the outcomes of treatment, that we know how long people will live, that my pain is the same as your pain, and that the QALY calculation can be carried out without difficulty and without assumptions.

(b) That in all cases where QALYS are used to discriminate it will be possible to calculate what to do. The idea that human beings are unique and have qualities that cannot be measured is not considered. Just as only a partial aspect of moral reasoning is recognized, it is assumed that all cases are, by and large, governed by the same few factors.

The selection of 'easy' cases as examples can help further this myth. For instance, if the choice lies between offering a life-saving course of treatment to a 35 year old man with a career and young family, or to help a 70 year old man with no close relatives, then QALYS help explain why it might at least make sense to discriminate against the older man if the treatment is scarce. However, it is a different matter if the choice is between a 13 year old boy and an 11 year old girl. If only one can be treated and the primary discriminatory measure—the length of expected life—is not applicable, and if all the other selected criteria are equal, then the QALY is of no help.

If a measure which makes claims to objectivity is to be used then it must be able to cater for all cases. But if it were to be applied in this case then not only is it shown to be inadequate as a measure, but it is also shown to disregard the principle of equal respect. The reason why it is morally difficult to discriminate between two children is that there is a deep feeling that these young people are entitled to equal respect and equal treatment. Why then are not the 35 year old and the 70 year old entitled to equal respect?

4. The slippery slope   It should now be obvious how easily the use and acceptance of QALYS could make it for us to slide down a slope where injustice to some can be 'justified' as being in the interest of the majority. This is the sort of justification that

Hitler used to explain his policy of murdering Jews (it was said to be in the interest of the German nation as a whole), and what the present government of South Africa uses to 'justify' apartheid. The claim is that 'everyone is better-off under this system than they would be under any other' (which assumes that everyone will agree about what 'better off'—the 'good'—means), and so this 'legitimizes' apartheid.

QALYS will inevitably discriminate on the ground of age, and they could easily be used to discriminate on the grounds of race, sex, or class. If you are old then your life expectancy is usually less than if you are young. Therefore, if there is to be a straight choice between the old and the young, the old must be sacrificed, regardless of how much they want to live, how much they have to give, or how much they value their own futures.

If you are a woman your life expectancy is longer than a man's, therefore you should receive the scarce resource—all other things being equal. But if you are a woman you might suffer from some medical conditions that men do not. If the treatment for these is more expensive than the treatment for his, and there is not enough money to go round, then you might find that you will not be treated, yet he will.

Epidemiological studies inform us that different races suffer from different diseases and have different life expectancies. So do the different classes. A member of parliament can expect a longer life then a mineworker, therefore, all other things being equal, the MP should be treated at the expense of the mineworker.

It does not require a major leap of imagination to understand how QALYS could be used to justify involuntary euthanasia, or the 'allowing to die' of severely handicapped infants, or the abandonment of mental patients who are no danger to society. Defenders of QALYS might argue that safeguards could be built into the system, and already exist within the legal system, but if so why not pick a better system in the first place?

The benefit of QALYS

The main benefit of the open discussion of QALYS is that they expose the implicit, though unintentional, injustice of some decisions that are taken in the present health service—injustice which might be avoided given a different structure and funding of the health service. QALYS remind us that health service resources are usually scarce not as a result of nature but as a result of a human decision to spend money elsewhere, for instance on nuclear weapons. And spending on nuclear weapons is usually 'justified' on the ground that they act to preserve human life by deterring warmongers. But the preservation of human life is a central role for the health service too, and in a more direct and obvious sense. Since war is not imminent there is a strong case that at least some of the military defence money be transferred to the health service which is constantly involved in the defence of human life.

What Should be Done?

As part of an argument against consequentialism and in support of the principle of justice, John Harris has proposed that the only fair way of distributing a scarce resource is to draw lots. Thus, if there are ten patients and only one bed in an intensive care unit then discrimination is not done with regard to the circumstances, instead a decision is made completely impartially and everything is left to chance. The person who draws the longest straw is the person to be saved! This is fair, but is it practicable? Would any doctor ever do this? It seems very unlikely. Also it does seem to offend against some commonly held moral intuitions that there must be very special circumstances if one person is to be treated rather than another.

We are now left with two unacceptable alternatives: to discriminate between people as a matter of policy—thus offending a basic principle of civilized society that all people are entitled to equal respect, regardless of their luck or their talents; or to be fair and draw lots for a scarce resource, which seems neither practical nor in accordance with the idea that there clearly are many cases where the drawing of lots is unacceptable. Randomness by itself does not amount to a policy of equal respect. How could a doctor explain to a mother that her young child had been sacrificed as the result of a lottery, to save an old man with only months left to live?

What is Needed is Experience, Consideration, and the Ability to Reason Morally

Sometimes hard choices have to be made. If a decision has to be made between who to treat and who not to treat then doctors do need some guidance. In some cases it might not be entirely immoral to treat the 15 year old rather than the 95 year old, or the 25 year old with a minor illness rather than the terminally ill 25 year old. A complete deliberation is necessary, of the type which will be enhanced by the use of the Ethical Grid. This deliberation might be made easier by work in teams.

Since each situation is unique the idea of applying a crude quantitative measure is inappropriate, and, what is worse, while trying to save the doctor from being stressed and feeling guilt the use of QALYS could turn her into a calculating machine. All she will have to do is measure simple differences, and she might begin to think that the computed answer is not her responsibility, but somehow objective, disregarding the fact that she has chosen to use the measure in the first place. What is needed is not an unjust technique but responsible, caring individuals and organizations—humane systems and not purely economic systems.

Two practical proposals

1. *That education in moral reasoning be given to all medical practitioners and health workers, on a regular basis*. That is, health workers should be given education in analysis of interventions, in weighing up strengths and weaknesses of alternatives by balancing them against each other, in the use of logic, in law, and in the assessment of duties and consequences.

    It should be explained that ethics is a process of deliberation in which it is necessary to select certain priorities from a range of possibilities. In any ethical deliberation in health work four levels should be addressed. These are external considerations such as evidence for one's judgement, duties, consequences, and the core rationale of health work. Consideration of the elements of the core will show clearly that the unqualified use of QALYS is simply not legitimate work for health. The use of QALYS will create autonomy in *some* individuals, it will respect the autonomy of *some* individuals, and it will serve *some* needs before wants but also some wants before needs; however, the use of QALYS certainly does not treat people with equal respect.

2. That since 'scarce resources' are scarce only as a result of lack of funds that might be available from other sources, and since by the use of statistics it is possible to predict fairly accurately how many dialysis machines and other such resources will be needed, *it should become public knowledge that lives are being lost and those doctors who must decide are being placed in impossible positions as a result of human priorities, not natural circumstances.*

Consequently there should be a recognized professional facility, whenever a health worker has to make a 'tragic choice'—sacrificing a life where that life could have been saved—for this to be publicly recorded. This could be done through the British Medical Association, who could ensure accuracy, and publicized each month in every national newspaper. Since newspapers regularly print stories of murder and road death as examples of avoidable injustice this should not be unappealing to them. It might even be desirable to have a league table of 'enforced injustice in medicine'.

In this way QALYS can work for good. If the measure ever does have to be used it should not be used on its own, without considering justice and unintended consequences, for instance. And it should not be seen as an objective rule. But if, in the hard world of medicine and health, the QALY measure does have to be a *part* of an assessment it should never be used in such a way as to legitimize discrimination, as if it is the only logical choice, as if it is the only moral choice, or as if it ought to be part of a true system of health care. It is not the only alternative and should not be used exclusively as part of a health service.

Conclusion

This chapter has outlined obstacles which might lie in the path of clear moral reasoning. Such obstacles should be avoided by health workers. If they are not overcome then it will not be possible to use the Ethical Grid.

Chapter Nine
The Background to the Ethical Grid

The Main Functions of the Next Two Chapters

Chapters Nine and Ten serve two main functions. They introduce step by step an important instrument to help health workers develop a powerful health work skill—the ability to reason morally. And, through this process of introduction and elucidation of the Ethical Grid, the many apparently disparate ideas contained in this book are pulled together.

An Analogy

The Ethical Grid is not a tool in the way that a conveyer belt is a tool, rather it is like a spade that a gardener will use to cultivate his land. The grid does not deliver 'the correct answer' in the way that a conveyer belt can be used to deliver neat packages.

Like a good gardener the proficient user of the Ethical Grid will understand the need to keep the tool as clean and as sharp as possible, and he will also know the best way in which to use the tool in order to get the best out of the situation, and in order that the material on which he is working will be treated in the best possible way. Whether the tool is a spade or the grid, and whether the tool is being employed on soil or persons, the good worker will appreciate when to use it since sometimes the conditions are not appropriate for the use of the tool—perhaps the ground will be waterlogged, or the law or a particular policy will be quite clear and agreed. And further, the end results of even the most proficient use of either of the tools are never entirely predictable. Even with the most conscientious practice there is no guarantee that the chosen method of digging (and there is a range of options open to gardeners) will produce the desired results in the plants, just as it is possible that even the most conscientious use of the grid may not produce the best practical results.

What Is the Grid, and How Does it Work?

On referring to the major figure (p. 141) the following features will be noticed:

1. There are four different layers to the grid which are indicated by different colours (blue, red, green, and black).

2. Each of the boxes, whatever its colour, is independent and detachable. However, although each box can stand independently all the boxes have strong relationships with one another.

3. The grid can be seen in more than one way. For instance, it is possible to use the grid as if the coloured layers have to be addressed in a particular order. So it might be considered that the most significant principles are those contained in the blue boxes at the centre of the grid, and that the outer boxes are of decreasing importance as one moves (or spirals if that is the method that is preferred) to the outer limit of the grid. But this use of the grid is not necessarily the most appropriate in all cases. It is even possible that some users of the grid will decide that this method is never one that they choose to use.

   As alternative legitimate options the user might choose to operate with a spiral running from the outer limit of the grid to the blue core, or she might always begin with a consideration of the consequences, say, or always consider—as a start—four particular boxes, one taken from each coloured layer.

   The grid can also be seen as either a two- or a three-dimensional object. If it is envisaged as a three-dimensional object then the four sides of the pyramid might each be considered in turn. However, it must be quite clear that *there is no special relationship or association between the boxes from the various layers that happen to fall together on each side of the pyramid*.

   Even if the grid is seen as a two-dimensional object it need not remain static on the page. It can be flexible in the imagination of the user. For instance, dependent upon the case in question and upon personal preference, it is possible to imagine that there is an invisible cord at the centre of the grid which can pull the grid (as if it were written on a piece of rubber) either towards or away from the viewer. The direction of the pull will depend upon the importance that the user wishes to accord to the various layers. In this way the grid can remain in view and in mind as a whole. It should be noted that this use of the grid has less flexibility than a use which regards each box as independent and detachable.

4. The grid has to be applied to practical cases in order for it to come to life.

Why is the Grid Composed of Different Coloured Layers?

First of all it must be explained that the grid is an artificial device, and that the separation of the boxes into apparently watertight compartments is also an artificial construction. It is not suggested that the ethical grid is an exact representation of the mental processes that make up moral reasoning. Moral reasoning is by no means as precise or neat as the grid might make it appear.

However, in order to provide health workers with a practical and accessible route into the complexity of moral reasoning, the layers have been separated out and distinguished by the use of colour. In time and with experience the grid might not need to be referred to at all—it should certainly never be believed to be a substitute for moral reasoning. However, even the most seasoned moral thinker might find it useful to refer back to the grid in order to be reminded of the various basic elements that need to enter into his deliberation.

And further, four distinct layers of the grid are shown in order to show that at least four different sets of elements make up comprehensive ethical deliberation. A deliberation which examines only the consequences of actions, or only the law, or only duties might happen to produce good results on occasions, but it will not be a deliberation carried through with integrity. And deliberations made in the context of health work should, if the actions which result are to be said to be health work at all, acknowledge at least one box from the blue layer.

It is not suggested that in each dilemma and before every intervention the health worker pulls out his 'pocket Ethical Grid'—his 'Health Worker's Guide to Life, the Universe and the NHS'—and selects boxes until he is satisfied that he has the right combination. This is clearly impractical. The benefits that are suggested are these: it is not claimed that the grid represents a new advance in ethical reasoning, but it does make some processes of moral reasoning more clear for those who are unfamiliar with this discipline. As such it is an aid both to understanding and to confidence. Thus the thoughtful health worker can become familiar with the grid and its use in the abstract, by practising on hypothetical cases, and by applying the grid to cases in practice (perhaps problems of management and resource allocation) where there is time. Proficiency in moral reasoning will improve in this fashion.

The Ethical Grid has been constructed with health professionals in mind, but it could also be used by people who are not paid to work for health. Work for health in its richest sense is work that every member of a society can be involved in.

The Blue Layer

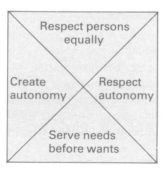

The blue layer is set at the centre of the grid since it provides the core rationale. The four boxes that make up the blue layer represent the notions that make up the richest idea of health. These boxes should not be thought to define health finally but, coupled with the theory that there are 'central conditions' necessary for health (see Seedhouse 1986, pp. 61–2), they present a rich and fruitful theory of health.

Without priority these boxes are: create autonomy, respect autonomy, respect persons equally, and act to serve needs before any other want.

Create autonomy

What is autonomy?

This question is addressed in more detail in a separate work (Seedhouse and Cribb 1988). However, it should be noted that personal autonomy refers to a person's capacity to choose freely for himself, and to be able to direct his own life. Autonomy is hardly ever pure but restricted by factors such as the law, social tradition, the autonomy of other people, and the prevailing circumstances of a person's life (for instance, the person's age, class, financial position, ambitions, and personality). Personal autonomy depends upon the possession of: the physical wherewithal to carry out one's chosen tasks (the environmental circumstances must also be suitable); a degree of knowledge sufficient to permit the person to pursue an end; an understanding of the routes open towards that end, the pitfalls, and the ways in which the knowledge can be employed in order to achieve that end; and the possession of an ability (sometimes referred to as the possession of rationality) to select ends appropriately for that person—for instance, if the person wishes to have a heart by-pass operation because he has been suffering from pains in his chest, yet the medical fact is that all he has is recurrent indigestion, then work is necessary to improve his ability to select appropriate goals.

Why is the creation of autonomy a part of the rationale of work for health? This question can be answered in two complementary ways: by focusing on the historical tradition of practice, and by studying the various legitimate abstract theories of health.

The historical tradition   Whatever the means, whether through a personal regime of living, or via medical and health professional intervention, practical work for health has always been carried out with the intention of creating autonomy. If treatments are not designed with this end in mind then there is very little point in making them at all—unless perhaps to make sure that a prisoner is fit to stand trial.

A broken arm is a physical impediment to autonomy, and is also an obstacle to biological development. A broken arm does not undermine individual autonomy completely—there will remain a wide range of individual choices and possibilities—but it does restrict a person's self-direction to a degree. The intervention to mend the broken arm is carried out in order to remove the obstacle to biological development, but this is not all; it is also carried out in order to enable the person to direct her own life again without the obstacle. The health intervention is done in order to allow the person the widest possible degree of autonomy. The whole point of humane treatment is to enable full persons to flourish as much as possible.

The principle of autonomy has, as a matter of fact, always inspired health work.

Theories of health all equate work for health, in some way, with the creation of autonomy

In a previous work (Seedhouse 1986) a variety of theories of health are presented and discussed. Among the most influential of these are the following: the theory that health is an ideal state (the option preferred by the World Health Organization), the theory that a person is healthy if he can function in a socially useful role, the theory that health can be bought or given as if it were a commodity, and the theory that health is an ability or a strength to adapt to the changing challenges and circumstances of life. Each of these legitimate theories of health incorporates the idea of autonomy to some degree. For instance, the World Health Organization's 'ideal state' is one in which a person is physically, mentally, and socially well, has a satisfying life, and can be economically productive. Although many of these terms are open to interpretation, a review of the WHO's literature makes it clear that a life cannot be satisfying without a level of autonomy. A degree of self-direction is necessary to carry out a socially useful role (although the degree required will vary dependent upon both the role and the society). The giving or selling of medical commodities (as discussed above) is done for a variety of reasons—sometimes a prime motivation is to make a financial profit—but it is valuable in direct proportion to the increased autonomy that is enabled in the receivers or purchasers of the commodities. The ability to adapt to the changing circumstances of life is actually a general definition of autonomy. According to this theory of health the primary goal—which might be achieved in countless ways—is the creation of personal autonomy, the creation of an ability to thrive and persevere whatever trauma is suffered.

Summary   A study of the practice and theory of health shows the extent to which autonomy is central to health work. The idea is such an abiding feature that it makes nonsense of claims that autonomy has no part to play in work for health. For instance, if for the sake of argument someone were to propose that health work has nothing to do with autonomy, and that the real aim of health work is to create *dependence*, it is hard to imagine how any meaningful discussion could actually begin. How can the removal of obstacles to the type of physical and mental potential which can enhance people's lives possibly be thought of as an attempt to create dependence?

Respect autonomy

The requirement to respect autonomy is a major part of the core rationale of health work, and it is significantly different from the necessity to create autonomy. The creation of autonomy requires the *provision* of the physical and mental wherewithal for rational (Seedhouse 1984; Seedhouse and Cribb 1988) self-direction, whereas respecting autonomy requires that the person's chosen direction should be respected, whether or not the health worker approves of that direction.

The box 'respect autonomy' raises an issue that is common in the field of *medical ethics*. That is, whether it is correct to respect the autonomy of individuals in *every* case. There are three main categories of problem. First, whether the autonomy of an individual should be respected if his choice will lead to harm only to himself—for instance, when a life-saving blood transfusion is refused by a person who is opposed to this practice on religious grounds. Secondly, whether the 'autonomy' of a person should be respected if there are strong grounds to suspect that the decision she has made has been made on belief that is false. For instance, if she refuses a course of treatment which will cure a condition on the ground that she has heard that it has terrible side-effects (and it does not), is deception about the treatment justifiable (can the same treatment be given to her under a different label)? And thirdly, whether the autonomy of a patient should be respected if his decision will lead to harm to other people. For instance, if a patient who has been diagnosed as carrying the AIDS virus informs his GP that he intends to carry on being promiscuous with as many partners as possible without informing them, should the GP respect this patient's autonomy? Further interesting questions arise in this context if the evidence for the different beliefs of doctor and patient is contested and not certain.

In the final case there is a clear need for the GP to balance the 'Respect autonomy' box with other boxes. He must certainly consider the consequences of any decision he might take, and he should draw on the boxes 'create autonomy' and 'respect persons equally' from the blue layer. It may be that his wish to respect persons equally overrides the impulse to respect one individual's autonomy in this case. However, in cases other than these difficult ones, which must be decided upon in context, it is an essential aspect of health work that autonomy should be respected. For example, if there is a range of treatments on offer, it falls to the health worker to explain this range and their effects (part of the process of creating autonomy), and then to respect the choice of the client, even if this choice is not what the health worker would have chosen for himself.

The idea of respecting autonomy is bedevilled with controversy. Many of the really hard cases in medical ethics hinge upon this principle, and whether or not it should be invoked in the context in question. Some of these controversies can be clarified with intelligent use of the grid, but there can be no final guidelines about how far individual autonomy ought to be respected. A very strong reason (although not abiding in all cases) not to respect individual autonomy is when the autonomous decision of the individual will harm one or more other people. Beyond this, the issues must be resolved by personal judgement and comprehensive and appropriate moral reasoning.

Respect persons equally

The requirement to respect persons equally when working for health follows from the requirement to create and respect autonomy in all people, and from the work by philosophers establishing basic criteria for personhood. We regard people as valuable not only because of what each person can do, but essentially because of what each person is. And the basic aspects of personhood—for instance, being able to value one's life, having the potential for future choices—are shared equally by all who are persons. The amount and type of future choices are bound to vary between individuals, but the potential for some rather than no future choices is a constant between persons. That choices exist at all means that some degree of autonomy must also exist.

The extent to which the box 'respect persons equally' is employed (which is another way of saying, 'the extent to which people are accorded equal respect') is dependent upon individual judgement. However, if this blue box is to be overriden by health workers, as with the other blue boxes, firmly convincing reasons will have to be given. If persons are not respected equally, perhaps because resources are scarce, then this is quite clearly *discrimination between beings who are fundamentally equal*. If such discrimination is seen to be condoned by a health service in a particular society for reasons that are not thoroughly justifiable then this must have dangerous implications for that society as a whole. What further discriminations then become justifiable?

Act to serve basic needs before any other want

This element of the core rationale of health work provides a natural grounding for the other three components. It gains its authority from the following sources: from the fact that a true health service must, before any other task, provide for the basic needs of all those it seeks to serve, and from the underpinning sense of 'justice as fairness'. For the reason that it is usually necessary to treat persons with equal respect it follows that it is necessary to ensure that all persons within a society have their basic needs met—so, if there are in a society people who have no shelter, or no food, or no purpose in life, or a very limited general education, while there are in the same society people whose material wants are being fulfilled then this is a system in which full health can never be achieved. And so this is a system in which there will be a lower degree of morality than there otherwise might be.

All human beings have needs that are part of a shared human condition. They are factual needs. 'Rights' vary over history and between contexts, and although it may be the case that through hard work some people deserve more benefits in life than those who do not work so hard, it is fundamentally unjust for any 'rights' and benefits to be enjoyed at the expense of the basic human needs. What is so important about medicine and health work is that this principle has always been acknowledged. In wartime medics do not (or should not) treat only the wounded from the army they are part of, and medical treatment is offered to criminals regardless of what crime they have committed. Within health work there is a basic humanizing principle. For example, if a hospital turns away one person with a broken leg whilst admitting another, on the ground that the first person is a bank robber and the second is a bank manager, then most people have little difficulty in recognizing that the action of the hospital is fundamentally wrong.

In summary

Create autonomy

Respect autonomy

(essential for the creation of full personhood)

Respect persons equally

(because of commonness of basic personhood)

Serve needs before wants

(because the *central conditions* of physical safety, knowledge, ability to act in life, purpose in life, and a sense of community are basic constitutents of health)

A review

Why are these boxes the core rather than any other boxes that could have been chosen?

The devil's advocate speaks again   'All that is going on in this writing about health—and now about ethics—is a fairly clever word game based on certain assumptions that you take for granted. *You* have decided what health is, and now, by the use of sophistry more than anything else, you attempt to deceive us into thinking that you are uncovering a conclusion. But you are doing nothing of the sort. All that is necessary to undermine your argument is to refuse to accept the assumptions you have chosen to accept, and to make alternative assumptions instead—perhaps premises that would be more acceptable to a person from a different political persuasion. For instance, it is just as valid to include these (or any other) boxes within the core 'health rationale': *manipulate clients, create dependency, discriminate between individuals according to their worth to a society as a whole, and act to provide a service for those who, through their own efforts, deserve the service, and do so before you pay any attention to the needy but undeserving.'*

The first response to this devil's advocate might be one of exasperation that he has not understood the logic of the argument of the book as a whole. The basic aim of the book is to provide a firm theoretical footing for a true health service, a health service which aims as its first priority to increase the degree of morality in the world through the interventions made in the name of health. Much of what has been said is connected as threads in a tapestry are connected. The threads begin and end in different places, but link together to bind the tapestry together and to present the best possible picture. Some of the threads that the devil's advocate should appreciate are these:

1. It has been shown that work for health has a common factor—namely the removal of obstacles to people's biological and intellectual potentials.
2. The associated ideas of enablement, personhood, and enhancing potential are (a) richer, more coherent and logically sound than the speculative alternatives of the advocate and (b) more likely to produce benefits that can be shared by all than any other option.
3. There is a clear relationship between ethics and health that has been demonstrated in these pages.
4. The Grand Thiam argument and the idea of dwarfing gives at least a strong indication that certain actions can be considered to be simply immoral. This further indicates that those features that might be the subject of dwarfing are precisely those which provide the basis for the equal treatment of all persons.
5. The existing rationale of health work—in theory and in practice—cannot be ignored. Although things could be better and priorities reassessed, the study of present health work practice shows that the principles outlined in the blue layer are those that inspire most health work.
6. The practical consequences are dreadful. How could a health service be organized according to the principles listed by the devil's advocate? Such a service would simply not be recognizable, and would not be a legitimate health service since although it would seek to remove some obstacles to some potentials, it would not do for all people equally, and some of the potentials could not be said to be enhancing potentials.

In deliberations, apart from the most exceptional cases, at least one blue box should be used. A decision not to use any needs a massive justification.

The Red Layer

This level of the grid is the level where the focus is placed upon duties and upon motive. What is it that the agent truly intends to do? The boxes included in this level are: promise-keeping, truth-telling, minimize harm, and beneficence (intent to

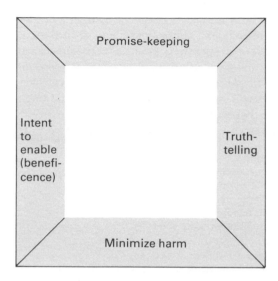

enable). The 'beneficence' box might appear to sum up the whole purpose of a health worker who makes use of the grid. However, although the idea which is the basis for the use of the grid is 'honestly seeking to enable the enhancing potentials of people', the 'beneficence' box does not go this far. It merely advises to do good rather than harm. Without the good being specified and defined this box is not ultimately powerful. Neither does the beneficence box include the notion of integrity, nor does it insist on the consideration of every layer of the grid.

What is the significance of this layer?

The red layer corresponds in the main with deontological theories of moral philosophy, in contrast with the green, consequentialist layer. The inclusion of this layer is to encourage the consideration of principles during moral deliberation. The principles of not doing harm, beneficence, promise-keeping, and truth-telling are not principles which should ever be dispensed with casually, although in practice from time to time instances will occur where it is better that they are temporarily disregarded and excluded from use. In all reflections about health work interventions it is important to bring these principles to mind, and if one, more, or even all are to be disregarded then very good reasons must be advanced.

The red layer is significant in the following ways:

1. In general

The principles of the red layer are less specific to health work practice than those of the blue layer, but they are intimately related to the richest sense of health. For instance, if one makes a promise to a person and then one proceeds to break it glibly, then one shows no respect. And respect is a central feature of health work.

2. The individual boxes

Beneficence   It has been argued that the principle of beneficence goes some way towards uniting deonotology and consequentialism. The thinking is that we do not seek to maximize good over evil simply because the consequences are better for most people, but because we actually have a duty to do good and to prevent harm—the principle of beneficence. The principle is called the principle of beneficence rather than the principle of benevolence because it makes the point that we should try in practice to do good and not evil, not merely that we should wish to do so.

Frankena has summed up the principle of beneficence in this way (Frankena 1963, p. 47):

> What does the principle of beneficence say? Four things, I think:
> 1) One ought not to inflict evil or harm (what is bad).
> 2) One ought to prevent evil or harm.
> 3) One ought to remove evil.
> 4) One ought to do or promote good.
>
> These four things are different, but they may appropriately be regarded as parts of the principle of beneficence. Of the four, it is most plausible to say that 4) is not a duty in the strict sense. In fact, one is inclined to say that in some sense 1) takes precedence over 2), 2) over 3), and 3) over 4), other things being equal. But all are, at any rate, principles of prima facie duty.

This has outlined the principle of beneficence in the abstract. To apply the principle one has to be quite clear about what counts as good and what counts as evil (see various parts of this book for analysis of this question). As it stands its main function is that of mnemonic.

Truth-telling   It may be that there are occasions on which it is better that the truth should not be told. And it may be that on occasions it is right that the truth is not told. But truth-telling is such an important principle of human conduct that a very strong justification is necessary if the principle is to be eschewed.

In the field of medical ethics there is a growing consensus that truthfulness is a central principle of conduct. Sometimes the principle may come into conflict with other principles (and must always be considered in terms of general consequences), such as not causing harm.

One major body in Britain at present which is out of step with this consensus is the British Medical Association. The Campaign for Freedom of Information has been campaigning since 1984 to give patients the right of access to their medical records, but at its annual conference in 1986 the BMA opposed access. The argument is that medicine is a technical subject which is difficult to communicate. However, in itself this is no reason not to try, and it suggests a need to spend more time and money on demystifying medicine and on researching ways of educating people better. It is also argued that no patient likes to hear depressing news, which is true, and that sometimes this truth might exacerbate their condition, which is more questionable. However, as Roger Higgs has pointed out (see Lockwood 1985), in no other walk of life would a professional consider it his duty to suppress information simply in order to preserve happiness. No accountant, foreseeing bankruptcy in his client's affairs, would chat cheerfully about the budget or a temporarily reassuring credit account. Yet such suppression of information occurs daily in wards and surgeries throughout the country. Higgs' argument is that if lies are to be told (and it is a lie to say 'I don't know' when one does) then there really must be no acceptable alternative. For Higgs the principle is the same as that which applies when the removal of someone's liberty is being considered under the Mental Health Act. When one considers telling a lie this is acting to remove or decrease a person's liberty, and we should view the action with precisely this degree of gravity.

Because of the enhancement of personal liberty that goes with learning the truth, because of the increase in autonomy, because of the implicit respect involved, truth-telling is an important principle in health work. If this box is to be dismissed during a deliberation in the name of health a very good explanation is required.

Minimize harm   It is better to remember to 'minimize harm' rather than 'do no harm' so far as medicine is concerned since surgery clearly inflicts injury (albeit sometimes for a greater good) and all medicines can be described as 'selective poisons'.

Not doing avoidable harm is a central principle of medical work. No health worker should intentionally wish to *dwarf* another individual in any way.

Although this is an important principle there may be occasions where short-term harm must be done to a person for the sake of a 'good' in the long run. For instance, a surgeon harms patients with his knife, but intends that they receive later benefit. And it may cause short-term harm to tell a person a painful truth, but this can be justified by reference to gains in the longer term.

Promise-keeping   Promise-keeping is a central duty. It is closely associated with the notion of respect for others. Many dilemmas in medicine centre on the principle of promise-keeping, especially with regard to issues of confidentiality. At what point should a doctor break a promise of confidentiality to his patient? The answer to this question can be found only in context. But promises should not be broken lightly. If health workers could not be relied upon to abide by their promises their integrity would be in question, and people would be discouraged from attending for help. Again, strong justification is necessary if this box is to be disregarded.

The Green Layer

The green layer divides up various aspects of the notion of consequentialism. Something has already been said about consequentialism (see p. 103). The green layer has been included as a separate layer in order to focus attention on the necessity always to consider the consequences of any proposed intervention. Not merely the immediate consequences ('If I do this then X will happen') but the consequences in general. Attention to the green layer will encourage reflection about whether the 'good' (to be specified in advance) is increased for humanity or a society as a whole, for a particular group (perhaps a disadvantaged group such as the handicapped, members of the black community, people living in a particular housing estate), for an individual, or for the agent himself. If the consequences of an action are an increase in the 'good' of the actor, and no one suffers as a result, then the action is moral in the terms of consequentialism.

As with the other layers and the grid as a whole nothing is clear-cut. It may be that all the boxes of the green layer can be brought into play, or it may be that only some can be used with others being redundant, or it may be that a box will have to be chosen

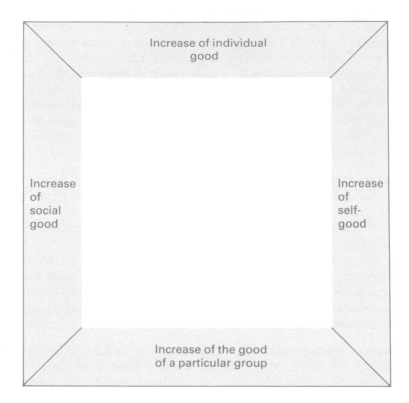

at the expense of other boxes. For example, when considering an intervention it might be concluded, having taken other factors into account, that in the interest of an increase in the social good, the good of a particular group might have to be sacrificed, or at least decreased. For instance, it is argued by politicians of the left that the group of people in the top 20 per cent of wage earners should pay more tax than they do at present in order that those who are less fortunate in society can enjoy better lives. It is argued that this redistribution of wealth will produce a general increase in the good of society as a whole. There will be less suffering, less resentment by the less well-off of the more wealthy, and less crime, for instance.

The importance of the green layer is best shown by the use of the grid.

The Black Layer

The black layer is of great importance, yet it includes factors that are often given insufficient attention by moral philosophers. The black layer is the level of external considerations. In many cases, in the real hard world, the black layer contains the most important factors of all. For instance, it may be that the legal rights of others, say to receive advice or a certain form of treatment, effectively takes the decision about what to do out of the hands of the health worker.

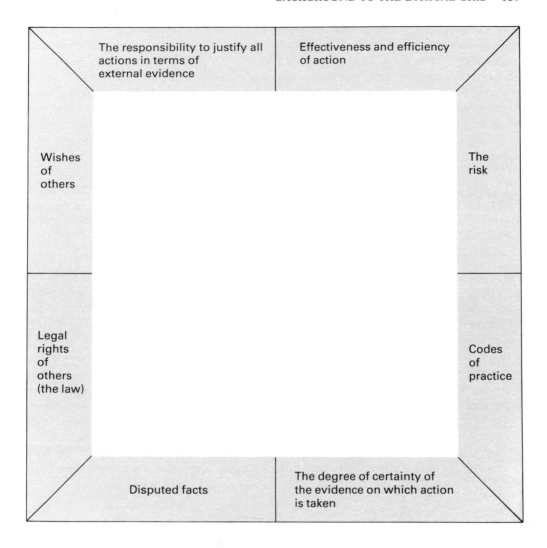

The responsibility to justify all actions in terms of external evidence

Effectiveness and efficiency of action

Wishes of others

The risk

Legal rights of others (the law)

Codes of practice

Disputed facts

The degree of certainty of the evidence on which action is taken

Ethics is not only a matter of deciding on principles, considering duties, and reflecting on likely outcomes in the abstract. Ethical intervention takes place in a world of limitations, a world which is always uncertain. Although it has been shown that law and morality do not necessarily correspond, the *law* that exists will have a clear part to play in the deliberation. However, in many cases the law is not a relevant factor. *Professional codes of practice*, although sometimes vague and imprecise, will have a bearing on the intervention. It is for the health worker to decide when, if ever, these codes are inadequate.

There is a necessity to assess the *degree of risk* of the intervention, in whatever sense is most relevant. Will physical harm occur? Is there a danger that an unfortunate precedent will be set? Is there a chance that the proposed intervention will produce unintended consequences? There is an associated demand on the actor to try to ensure that whatever intervention is made is carried out with the *maximum efficiency and effectiveness*.

It is also necessary to consider the *degree of certainty of the evidence* on which the action is taken, and to take account of those facts of the matter that are clear and undisputed. Not to do so would, by any standard, be foolish. It is also very important not only to 'respect people' in the abstract, but to ascertain *what their wishes are* in practice. Since most professional health workers are in a position of some power, and have a degree of status, many clients may be overawed, and may have decisions imposed on them, even if the imposition is unwitting. Health workers should in every case try to clarify the wishes of those they are trying to help, and of those other people who care for them and are affected by what happens to them, and should try to help them conceive of their position and choices as plainly and accurately as possible.

Finally, *one black box should be used on all occasions*. There is an abiding responsibility on anyone who intervenes in the life of another person to be able to *justify all actions in terms of the external evidence*. Any person who has reasoned morally in a proper fashion will be in an excellent position to do this.

The Limit to the Grid

The limit to the grid is quite straightforward. It can be used legitimately only by those who *honestly seek to enable the enhancing potentials of people*; by those who do not suffer from bad faith. In other words the grid can be used legitimately only by those who are consistently opposed to *dwarfing*, and devoted to the fight against it (*dwarfing* can mean either the deliberate attempt to diminish people, or any diminishing which is avoidable). Consequently the grid can be used only by people with integrity. If it is used insincerely, if the grid is employed cynically—merely to get the best results in order to further some personal goal, for instance—then this is not a moral use, even though the outcomes might not be significantly different from those resulting from sincere use. The need for integrity inevitably places a clear onus on all health workers to recognize a basic responsibility for all the decisions they take and interventions they make.

A Claim for the Grid, and What it Cannot Do

The Ethical Grid is a tool, and nothing more than that. Like a hammer or a screwdriver (used competently) it can help make certain tasks easier, but it cannot direct the tasks, nor can it help decide which tasks are the most important.

It is perhaps unfair to compare the grid with a hammer since it has a far wider range of functions. Contained within the grid is a substantive theory of both health and morality, which is explained in the rest of this book. The grid can be used in different ways, but not like a calculator or a slide-rule. There can be very few certain answers in moral reasoning. Everything depends upon the judgement of the person who is deliberating. The grid can enhance this deliberation, it can throw light into unseen corners, and it can suggest new avenues of thought—but *the grid is not a substitute for personal judgement*. To think of the grid in these terms would be a gross misunderstanding.

It should not be thought sufficient for moral reasoning merely to select boxes at random, through habit, or without thought about the implications of the selection. True moral reasoning requires personal involvement. It is an essentially human activity which touches sensitive nerves and frequently exposes raw frailty.

The Ethical Grid can improve moral reasoning but it cannot take its place. Responsibility lies with the user and not with the grid. The grid is not a model of the psychology of moral reasoning. It is not all there is to moral reasoning. In ethical reflection much depends upon the personal capacity, preferences, and mode of thought of each individual, and these aspects simply cannot be properly presented graphically.

This is illustrated by the fact that reflection about each separate box reveals that each box can be interpreted in such a way that it *contains* all the other boxes. In other words, if one box is taken on its own, say 'create autonomy', inevitably all the other factors listed in the grid will have to be considered, at least in general. To take a box on its own, without considering the boxes in the other layers, is both hollow and impractical.

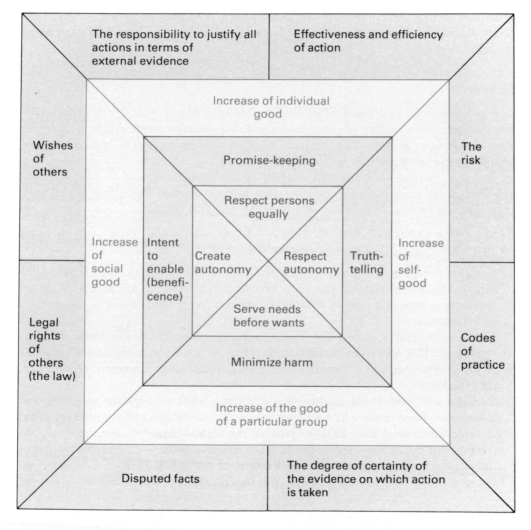

The limit to the use of the grid is that it should be used honestly to seek to enable the enhancing potentials of people.

Chapter Ten
The Use of the Ethical Grid

The Recommended Use of the Ethical Grid

There are various possible uses of the Ethical Grid. The manner of use preferred depends ultimately on the person who is to use the grid. However, the following use is recommended.

In general

It is recommended that the Ethical Grid be brought into play at every opportunity. For instance, when reading of moral issues in newspapers, or when watching television documentaries, or when reading literature, or when considering friends' problems in life, or when considering the way in which one deals with situations in one's own life. It is important to practise with the grid in order to see its nuances, and to understand its possibilities and limitations. Proficiency comes with experience. The ultimate goal for a person should be to gain sufficient skill to render the grid obsolete.

In practice

1. Consider the issue intuitively, without reference to the grid. Try to understand the extent of the ramifications of possible action. Clarify the issue by key aspects. Attempt to list basic pros and cons of the various options for action. Arrive at an intuitive initial position.
2. Consider the grid. Consider first the layer which is intuitively felt to be the most significant. This will often be the blue layer since this layer contains the rationale of work for health, and no genuine health work intervention can ignore every box of the blue layer.
3. Consider all other levels of the grid, selecting—after appropriate weighing and balancing—those boxes which appear to offer the most appropriate solution. That is, those which seem most likely to produce the highest degree of morality.
4. Arrange the boxes 'over' the dilemma. That is, apply them to the mental picture of the proposed intervention. In this way a course of action will have been decided, and the means to justify it in moral terms will be available.

Two Case Studies Considered with the Use of the Ethical Grid

Since the grid cannot produce 'right answers' as a calculator can produce 'right numbers' it is possible for different people to use the grid on the same issue and arrive at different solutions. It falls to individuals to justify their solutions and select the option which produces the highest degree of morality.

1. Teaching or caring: Michael and Caroline

Michael is the empathic health visitor. As part of his training he was assigned an elderly widow called Caroline. Although no specific nursing role was necessary Michael visited Caroline once a month for eight months and the two became friends. Both Caroline and Michael were benefiting in different ways from the friendship.

After this period Michael qualified, at which point his superior assigned him a different case load, even though he was still operating the same patch. Michael's supervisor explained that Caroline's circumstances did not really merit the services of a busy health visitor, and that the old lady had been useful only as part of Michael's learning experience. Michael accepted this reasoning reluctantly, but responded that he would, in this case, continue to visit Caroline in a private capacity. But his supervisor forbade even this, arguing that it would be a 'very unprofessional' action.

Different intuitions

Clearly different intuitions are possible about this case. In order to discover the most ethical intervention(s) possible it is appropriate to scrutinize the intuitions with the use of the Ethical Grid.

The intuition of health worker A   It is felt by this health worker that there is something about the supervisor's treatment of both Michael and Caroline that is profoundly wrong. It seems that Michael and Caroline, in their own ways, both wish to enable each other— not solely as a means of furthering their own self-interests, but in a way that respects the individuality of the other. It is suspected that the supervisor has a hidden motive. Perhaps she feels that Michael's activities, and his success, pose a threat to her power and authority.

Intuitively, health worker A believes that the following proposal creates the highest degree of morality. Since two people will benefit Michael should—to carry out the most ethical intervention—ignore the wishes of his supervisor, and continue to visit Caroline whilst at the same time performing a responsible and caring role with his new case load. (Health worker A has chosen to focus on Michael's possible interventions since he is seen as the central character.)

The intuition of health worker B   It is felt by this health worker that there is something far too impulsive about the way in which Michael is behaving, and she also has a gut feeling that the overall interests of the other people who work as health visitors, as well as those who are visited by the health visiting profession, will not be served by the supervisor approving of Michael's request, or by her turning a blind eye to his visits to Caroline.

Michael and Caroline are mavericks, rebels who unintentionally threaten to disrupt the smooth running of a system which—in the way it operates at present, according to rules, codes, hierarchies, and established principles—operates to serve the best interests and needs of the community as a whole.

Health worker B focuses on the supervisor as the central character. According to this health worker the most ethical form of intervention that the supervisor can make is to insist, in strong terms, that Michael obeys her request as behoves a professional. This is not seen as a callous action. Michael's feelings and future as a good health visitor are taken into account. It is felt that this intervention is in Michael's best interest. The supervisor should, in addition to her reprimand, see to it that Michael receives proper counselling, in-service training, and even career guidance if he cannot bring himself to accept the decision.

Health worker B is convinced that Caroline is perfectly capable of looking after herself, and should not be a burden on public funds. She believes that neither the public interest nor Caroline's interest will best be served by her continuing a relationship that began, and should have remained, as one between health visitor and client. In the opinion of this health worker a continuing relationship will not be good for Caroline or Michael, and it will not be good for Michael's other clients since the relationship could interfere with his professional responsibilities and relationships with clients in genuine need.

(Other intuitive positions will inevitably occur. However, for the sake of clarity the analysis is restricted to two.)

The grid in use

Once the key factors have been listed by the health workers the grid can be brought into service. It may be that the grid will confirm the initial intuition, lending it substance and intellectual credibility, or it may be that the use of the grid will actually lead to a change of mind by the health worker. In either case the use of the grid will be of great value.

A possible use of the grid by health worker B   Health worker B, who has integrity and who is honestly seeking to enable the enhancing potentials of individuals, is drawn immediately to the green layer of the grid. After reflection on the key factors of the case (she regards these as 'professional responsibility', 'the public interest', 'respect for authority', and 'the maintenance of codes of practice') she believes that the overriding consideration should be the long-term consequence of the supervisor's intervention. She feels that if the supervisor insists that her instructions must be obeyed then the consequences for the individuals concerned will be better—Michael especially will benefit—and that the consequences for society as a whole will be better because health visiting must be seen to operate according to certain standards.

Health worker B, using the grid properly, considers the other layers of the grid. She feels that although the *autonomy* of Michael and Caroline *is not being respected*, and that by not giving him a free hand in his private life *no further autonomy is being created* in Michael, people are being *respected equally* by the supervisor (no exceptions are being made), and *needs are being served before wants* (Michael wants to see Caroline who has no need—his time could be better spent serving the needs of others).

The red layer is considered and it is concluded that the *truth is being told*, that *no harm is being done*, and that a positive good—in the long term—is being produced. A similar analysis is carried out on the black layer and the health worker's judgement remains the same.

A possible use of the grid by health worker A   For health worker A the starting point is not the green layer but the blue core. His analysis runs in this manner.

He decides to consider each blue box in turn, to see how it relates to the case in question. He begins with the box 'create autonomy'. What is clear is that the autonomy of both Michael and Caroline is being impeded by the decision taken by the supervisor. The requirement to create autonomy by removing obstacles from people's physical and intellectual paths, to enable them to take greater charge of their own destinies, is a central principle of health work. The issue is whether the impairment of two people's autonomy can be justified, either by pointing to greater future gain in autonomy, or by showing that the beliefs and wishes of Michael and Caroline are somehow deficient.

In this case the ideas of creating autonomy and respecting autonomy are not far apart. Unless their beliefs can be shown to be clearly mistaken in some way it cannot be denied that the choices of Michael and Caroline are not being respected, but overridden by authority.

On considering the box 'respect persons equally' it becomes clear to health worker A that this is the key consideration. A strong case can be made out that neither Michael nor Caroline are being afforded the basic respect due to persons. Caroline in particular is being abused. To use Kant's terminology, Caroline is being used as a means rather than an end. She is not being treated as a person but as an object. She has been used as a means by which to train the health visitor. Her personal circumstances and needs are immaterial, all that is necessary is that somebody should be available so that Michael can learn and develop health visiting skills.

And Michael, too, is not being respected as a person, as a unique individual—a unique world. All that matters is that one more efficient, rule-following, functional health visitor is trained. Health worker A is clear that work for health is not merely work directed against disease and illness, and that work for health is not only work to create health in a patient but in all those involved in an intervention. With this in mind he concludes, provisionally, that the supervisor's action has offended against a vital principle. On limited evidence health worker A also concludes that it is likely that Caroline does have needs which Michael can meet.

Having considered the blue layer, the next stage for the health worker is to consider the other layers, and to be prepared to reassess his provisional conclusions made during his analysis of the blue core if necessary. The most appropriate layer on which to focus might be the black level, the level of external considerations. What laws might come into play? Could the supervisor act to punish Michael if he continued to see Caroline privately? This is unclear. Michael would certainly not be breaking any criminal or civil law, but the supervisor might attempt to initiate internal disciplinary procedures on the ground of 'unprofessional behaviour'. Would such a course of action be likely? Can it be clearly established that Caroline does, in fact, have needs which justify health visitor support? Or is Michael actually being self-indulgent. What are the motives and goals of the three people involved? How genuine is Michael?

After establishing as much as possible about the external circumstances health worker A should consider the red and green levels, in as much depth as is considered appropriate. Is the principle of beneficence being offended against? What are the likely consequences of the various courses of action? The health worker does not spend too long on these layers in this context on the grounds that the principles of the blue core are primary, because the consequences are unclear, and whatever they might be they will not be of any significant import except to Michael, Caroline, and the supervisor. Since this is the judgement of the health worker he concludes that Michael should disobey the supervisor, explaining his reasons to her, and should continue with his mutually beneficial relationship with Caroline. He selects the following boxes to apply to the case: *respect persons equally*, *increase of individual good*, *beneficence*, and the *justification of actions in terms of external evidence*.

Analysis

Which of the proposals of the two health workers is the most convincing? Which will produce the highest degree of morality?

Both health workers have deliberated with integrity. Both have used the grid legitimately, yet they have produced conflicting responses. For one the supervisor is justified in her action while the other recommends that she be disobeyed. A case can be made out for both responses, however health worker A's position is more in tune with the rationale of work for health, and suggests an approach that will *increase morality to a higher degree*.

This conclusion cannot be demonstrated with certainty. As events unfold it might even turn out that health worker B's proposal would have been far more satisfactory. But one can judge only on what seems likely at the time, on what evidence is available, and in accordance with whatever principles are espoused. Because health worker A's proposal shows respect for the individuals involved, because a genuine attempt is made to enable those concerned directly, also taking into account the likely outcomes in the long term, and because proper attention is paid to the potentials of all concerned rather than reference to some unspecified 'social good' (and it is not clear how this 'good' is to be created by the supervisor's hard line), health worker A's proposal appears to produce a higher degree of morality in direct proportion to the amount of enhancing potentials enabled in Michael and Caroline.

2. Sponsorship and hidden motives

The second example of how to use the grid has been chosen because of its reality, and because opinion can be clearly split into two camps (although there is a range of proposals in between). The issue is this: What is the most ethical intervention possible from the standpoint of the professor?

Professor Ronson is head of a Department of Community Medicine. He wants his department to be involved in as many research projects which will benefit the community as possible. He also wishes to employ as many research staff as possible since he appreciates that, because of short-sighted government economies, it is becoming increasingly difficult for researchers to find posts at universities and polytechnics. Professor Ronson has an idea for a research project to discover the reasons why there is a relatively low use of the medical and health facilities, which include a health centre and a well-women's centre, in one part of the city. The uptake rate was expected to be fairly low because the area in question is the poorest in the district, with the highest levels of unemployment and single-parent families, and such areas usually produce low rates. However, the reasons for the lack of use of the facilities are not known. Taking into account the fact that the local population suffers a disproportionately high level of disease and illness it seems to be unquestionably important to understand more about why the people act as they do.

Professor Ronson has exhausted his research budget so he makes it known to potential sponsors and research bodies that he wishes to embark on a two-year project, employing at least one research associate. Unfortunately for the professor, none of the usual sources of funds wishes to or is able to help. However, out of the blue there comes an offer of sponsorship from a famous tobacco company. The company tells Professor Ronson that it intends to fund worthwhile health research throughout the country and is pleased to say that this is one of its first offers. The dilemma is clear: should Professor Ronson accept sponsorship from a company which trades in a commodity which creates disease and illness.

Another way of expressing the issue is to ask what is the most ethical form of intervention that the professor can make. Although there is no direct intervention into the life of another person in this case, the repercussions of doing either something or nothing must indirectly affect the lives of other people. Eventually there may be direct and dramatic effects.

Two contrasting intuitions

Once the key features have been identified very different perceptions are possible.

The intuition of health worker C   This health worker decides 'instinctively' that Professor Ronson should not accept the money from the tobacco company. Such an action would be entirely unprincipled, it would undermine the whole ethos of the health service, it would reflect great discredit on Professor Ronson, and it would provide a valuable source of propaganda for the tobacco industry. The tobacco companies would, if their sponsorship were to be accepted, be able to advance the claim that they were being endorsed by the health service.

The intuition of health worker D   Even though it occurs to health worker D that many people will feel that there is something intuitively offensive about a sector of the health service accepting money from a tobacco company, she does not regard this as being of crucial importance. On reflection she sees that there is much to be gained by accepting the sponsorship rather than turning it down. More people will benefit if Professor Ronson accepts the money.

After all, the health service is funded from a source that is arguably more reprehensible than the tobacco companies. The State or the government of the day is by far the largest sponsor of the health service. And it can be said of the State that much of what it does actually harms the health (in a medical sense as well as in other senses) of the population. For instance, the government permits industrial pollution, it manufactures nuclear weapons which might be used, and it allows people to suffer unemployment when, with alternative policies, it could ensure full employment. Yet apparently no one has any qualms about accepting funds from this source, and then putting them to good use.

The use of the grid in this case

It falls to each health worker to consider each level of the grid in some order, either to justify the initial intuition or to appreciate the merits of an alternative.

The use of the grid by health worker C   It is most likely that the starting point on the grid for health worker C will be either the green or the red layer. Probably, a person inclined against acceptance of the offer of sponsorship will justify her position in accordance with certain principles, with regard to the likely consequences, or both. Health worker C might consider that, taking into account as much external evidence as possible, if Professor Ronson accepts then the overriding factor will be that the balance of good over evil for society as a whole will be substantially decreased. Even if there will be an increase of good over evil for the professor, for the research associate, for the university, and for the disadvantaged section of the population, this is outweighed by the increased credibility given to the tobacco companies.

On the red level there is a duty incumbent on the professor to minimize harm, and health worker C considers that to accept the offer will, indirectly, lead to harm. This health worker is convinced that the intent of the tobacco company is not altruistic but that it is seeking propaganda, and also it needs evidence that it can do good works to help in its fight against measures to curtail its business. On considering the blue level, health worker C thinks that the intervention is too indirect to raise issues of autonomy, respect, and justice.

The professor should decline the sponsorship. The boxes *minimize harm*, *increase of social good*, and *justify actions in terms of external evidence* are regarded as of most significance.

The use of the grid by health worker D   Health worker D also begins with the layer of consequences. However, this health worker considers that the good consequences for the professor, the university, the disadvantaged group, and the research associate, outweigh the possible decrease in the social good. After reflecting on the black layer the health worker reasons that the effect on society as a whole is so open to speculation that the probable outcome of the professor's acceptance of sponsorship can be no more than a matter of opinion. It is just as likely that the outcome of a fine research project could produce significant nationwide benefits for similar groups of people, and that direct and clear improvements in the quality of life of many people could result. There is no evidence that this benefit would lead to more people smoking, nor is it certain that the tobacco company's efforts (whatever its motive) will prevent legislation curtailing their marketing activities.

The health worker considers that the beneficence box is the most relevant on the red level. She also thinks that the blue core is very relevant. She believes that a successful research project could lead to significant increases in the autonomy of the disadvantaged individuals, and will certainly enhance the scope and self-direction of the research associate, whilst even if there are spin-offs for the tobacco company these will not reduce general levels of autonomy.

Professor Ronson should accept the money, and denounce smoking at the same time if that is what he wishes. The boxes *create autonomy*, *increase of self-good*, *increase of individual good*, *increase of the good of a group*, *beneficence*, and *justify actions in terms of external evidence* are regarded as of most significance.

Analysis

Objectivity is not possible in ethical deliberation but in my opinion the appropriate analysis has already been carried out. For the reasons advanced by health worker D the professor should accept the money in order to create a higher degree of morality.

Chapter Eleven
Implications

This chapter is short. The implications of the analysis of this book for the future of health care are immense. A wide range of futures are possible, but for a strong indication of how the future might be it is wise to look at practice, and the investigation of practice is beyond the scope of this book. There is, however, a complementary volume in this series (*Changing Health Care*, Seedhouse and Cribb 1988), which is concerned with precisely this sort of empirical inquiry, and which addresses the implications which stem from present practice. Where *The Ethics of Health* begins with theory and moves to consider practice, *Changing Health Care* begins with practice and moves on to reflect upon the importance of the practices discussed for the development of theories of health care. *Changing Health Care* might be seen as an annexe to this chapter, although it is much more than this.

The pages of this book are mainly the result of reasoning in the abstract, reasoning done by a person trained as a philosopher. But this does not mean that the value of this reasoning can be assessed only in the abstract. In this book philosophy—a process of clarification—has been applied to a general problem of practice; namely, *How can health work be developed into a more moral endeavour*? Although answers to questions such as What is health? and What is ethics? do have to be assessed at first in the abstract, the answer to this general problem of practice has to be practical too. Better practical answers cannot come about simply as the result of more practice, but are formed from a combination of clarification, analysis, logic, and application of theory to practice.

There exists an unfortunate habit among some sorts of people of labelling other individuals with a single title which is then thought to describe every aspect of that person. Such behaviour is a further form of *bad faith*, where others are labelled as objects, as fixed essences. It should be noted that simply because a person happens to have had a philosophical training, and frequently advocates the merits of philosophy, this does not mean that he is solely a philosopher. He can also be a gardener, a decorator, a heavy drinker, a teacher, a cultural philistine, a health educator, and a rogue. As such he will be about as well qualified as any other reasonably practical person to understand and discuss practical problems.

At the end of Part I of the book the following abstract issues were outlined: How can we work towards health when we are not clear about what health is? How can we be more ethical when we are not sure what 'being ethical' means? What limits should there be to interventions? Which sorts of intervention are legitimate interventions in the name of health, and which are not acceptable? What is a person? What are human beings for?

Substantial progress has been made with all these issues. The nature of health has been clarified in an earlier work, and in these pages its nature has become clearer still. It is now apparent that work for health is actually a moral endeavour. It is not a moral endeavour in the sense that a particular, specifiable good is being pursued. Rather it is an endeavour which seeks to produce a higher degree of morality in the world by trying to enable as many enhancing potentials as fully as possible during health work interventions.

Such interventions seek to create more 'full persons'—in other words more fulfilled people—in the world. Rich health work interventions are opposed to *dwarfing*, which is the intentional or accidental limiting of people. Rich health work interventions should be attempted with integrity, with the aim of honestly seeking to enable the best possible state of affairs for people. This is the theoretical limit to health work. Work which is not done in this spirit of honesty is not legitimate health work.

Since 'full persons' are not only physical beings but have complex mental lives the intellect and the emotions are also targets for health work. Because of this, and because of the fact that 'persons' are fundamentally equal, the principles of 'respect for autonomy', 'equal respect for persons', 'create autonomy', and 'serve needs before wants' can now be seen to be at the very heart of health work theory and practice.

What might the practical implications of the rather complicated theoretical analysis of this book be?

Possibilities

If the above principles (the principles which form the core of the Ethical Grid) are taken seriously, if they are recognized as basic to health work, then priorities must shift. If these principles are given precedence then the ways in which people think about the nature of health care will change radically. For instance, although morbidity and mortality statistics and epidemiological research will always play an important part in the provision of effective health care, they will not remain as exemplars of the primary *raison d'être* of health care. If, for example, the principle of 'respect autonomy' is placed above the duty 'always to preserve life' present taboos might become respectable. It might become the case that doctors and carers enable people in terrible pain, and with no prospect of recovery, to end their lives if that is what they wish. And if the principle of 'create autonomy' gains prominence then far more emphasis will be placed upon educating people rather than merely treating their bodies with some technique or other. Indeed, many current practitioners regard the process of education as a vital and valuable treatment in itself. And if the idea of 'equal respect for persons' is acknowledged to be a central principle then such discriminatory devices as QALYS will simply be unacceptable unless they are used as part of a moral process involving other types of deliberation.

These are only three possible major changes among an indefinite number of possibilities that will occur to different health workers.

One Possibility—a Modern Peckham

In 1935 a 'pioneer health centre' was built in Peckham in South London (Pearse 1985). The centre was designed and intended to be for the use of local families, who were predominantly working class. The idea was for the members to choose for themselves how the building was to be run, within a given structure. The building consisted of a swimming pool, consulting rooms, reception rooms, a caféteria, a recreation room and a day-nursery. The centre was intended to be a comfortable place offering the atmosphere and shared facilities of the kind provided by village halls and greens in previous decades and in rural areas.

The facilities offered by the Peckham health centre were as follows: antenatal clinic; postnatal clinic; birth control clinic; infant welfare clinic; care of the toddler; nursery school; immunization service; schoolchildren's medical examinations; vocational guidance; sex instruction for adolescents; youth centres; sports clubs and recreation clubs of various kinds; keep fit and gymnastics classes; adult education; music, debates, drama, and any event agreed by the members; citizens' advice bureau; holiday organizations; outings and exhibitions; a bar; billiards; dancing; social gatherings; a marriage advice bureau; a child guidance clinic; a poor men's lawyer; a social worker; and a rehabilitation clinic.

In 1951 the health centre was forced to close through lack of money.

The importance of the background rationale

The development of health centres such as Peckham throughout the country, which would provide a modern comprehensive caring service within a single unit, is one possible future development in line with the richest sense of health. Such health centres—and, equally, any of a great range of other possible improvements—would be supported by a changed background system. Such a system would insist on educating all health workers in a wider range of enabling skills—including education in the ethics of health care as a necessity rather than a peripheral activity. It would eschew intense and divisive hierarchies; it would advocate a vastly developed notion of health education; it would incline towards the demystification of medicine; and it would announce and stand by a clear declaration which acknowledged the basic principles of health care—principles which would be known to all users of the service. The existence of this background rationale would help dismantle the practical barriers between the various types of health worker. And people who have not seen their work as health work, people such as lawyers, counsellors, and youth workers, would be able to regard themselves as health workers too.

The point of briefly describing Peckham is not that this is the ideal, or that a system of 'Peckham health centres' is the only possible form for a health service cast in the spirit of the new paradigm. It is discussed merely to show that other structures for health care are possible, and can be far more comprehensive—and enable people better—than services controlled by medicine. For instance, if the goal of a health service is held to be solely the prevention of physical and mental disease then it is still quite in order for a health centre to provide a readily accessible legal aid solicitor. There has been much research evidence to support the proposition that stress can cause both mental and physical disorders. And it is also well known that lack of sound legal advice can create stress. A further example of how readily available legal assistance can be seen as work for health as disease prevention concerns housing. If a family occupies a cold damp house they are more susceptible to some diseases, including bronchitis. If the local council is contacted about the poor living conditions by the family alone then their complaints may carry little weight, and they may not be familiar with the correct complaints procedure. Legal assistance can speed up the process and might perhaps result in a family being rehoused where they would not have been had they pursued the task independently.

What About Resources?

An obvious objection to such visions is that they are 'pie in the sky', and that the funds for them are just not available in the real world outside the speculations of philosophy. Whether or not the money exists is a matter for empirical research. Certainly a vast amount of money is spent on military defence whilst the defence of personal health is not such a priority.

The ways in which the national budget is spent are not somehow preordained. The decisions taken about what money is spent where are made by human beings. And just because someone with particular values has decided that there is only a specific limited amount of money available for health care this does not mean that other people cannot campaign for more, or that it is wrong or unrealistic to do so.

Even if the present 'health budget' is all that is possible, interventions within the scope of this budget can be made in a way designed so as to increase the level of morality in the world. From these practical changes to increase morality within the confines of a budget a restructuring of services, and the ways in which those services are given, can follow. By changing the form of health care, even if in only apparently minor ways such as always being friendly and informative when you write and hand out prescriptions, the very objectives of health care are also affected. Over time, attempts at empathy and understanding in consultations will become part of what work for health is all about.

If one achievement in the philosophy of health has to be stated it should be this. For some years theorists and health professionals of many kinds have been aware that work for health is more, must be more, than work set against disease and illness. However, the nature of the wider target of work for health has been vague at best. There has been a real feeling that work for health should 'enable' and be 'positive' and be 'enhancing' but, without clarification and thorough background thinking and theory, these terms must remain nebulous and open to wide interpretation. 'Positive well-being' might be exactly the same thing as 'enhanced marvellousness', but without definition of these terms based on logical and coherent theory they are empty jargon. It might just as well be said that 'we are not only working against disease but we are working for goodness, and a lot of it'! This book has shown quite clearly that there are extensive problems of value conflict associated with working towards some ill-defined 'good'.

But now there is true substance through which to develop meaningful targets for work for health. This work in the philosophy of health has presented principles, such as 'create autonomy', and has associated work for health with the endeavour to be moral. Together these ideas allow health workers a clear and practical base on which to strive for health in a richer sense.

Since work for health is a moral endeavour, since health work is a fight to bring out the fullest possible latent human capacities regardless of age or sex or race, then it is truly the most civilizing task that mankind can follow. What other enterprise could be so universal and so egalitarian?

And if those with power in a society espouse other priorities then it falls to each of us, to each thinking and caring person, to shout '*Why*?' Why is it that you choose to dwarf us when you could increase our health? How dare you deny me a fulfilled life? How dare you limit what I could be? How dare you *dwarf* me?

References and Further Reading

Archambault, R.D. (1966) *Dewey on Education: Appraisals*. Random House, New York.

Aristotle (1976) *Ethics*. Translated by J. A. K. Thomson. Introduction by J. Barnes. Penguin.

Ashton J. R. (1984) *Health in Mersey—A Review*. University of Liverpool Medical School, Department of Community Health.

Ashton, J. R., Grey, P., and Barnard, K. (1986) 'Healthy cities—WHO's new public health initiative', *Health Promotion*, **1** (3), 319–24.

Black, D., Townsend, P., and Davidson, N. (1982) *Inequalities in Health: The Black Report*. Penguin.

BMA (British Medical Association) (1984) *The Handbook of Medical Ethics*. British Medical Association.

Brennan, J. G. (1973) *Ethics and Morals*. Harper & Row.

Dewy, J. (1920) *Reconstruction in Philosophy* (1920, New York, New American Library 1950).

DHSS (Department of Health and Social Security) (1986) *Neighbourhood Nursing—A Focus for Care*. Report of the Community Nursing Review (The Cumberledge Report). HMSO.

Dobson, C., and Miller, J. (1982) *The Falklands Conflict*. Hodder & Stoughton.

Edwards, P. (1972) *The Encyclopedia of Philosophy*. Macmillan.

Ellis, W. D. (ed.) (1938) *A Source Book of Gestalt Psychology*. London.

Emmet, D. (1979) *The Moral Prism*, Macmillan, London.

Frankena, W. K. (1963) *Ethics*. Prentice-Hall.

Gardner, K. (1983) 'A well-woman clinic in an inner city general practice', *Journal of the Royal College of General Practitioners*, November.

Goldthorpe, G. E. (1985) *An Introduction to Sociology*. Cambridge University Press.

Greaves, P. (1979) 'What is medicine? Towards a philosophical approach', *Journal of Medical Ethics*, **5**, 29-32.

Gruber, H.E., Voneche, J.J. and Piaget, J. (1977) *The Essential Piaget*, Routledge & Kegan Paul, London.

Gullin, J. I., and Franci, A. S. (1985) *AIDS*. Raven Press.

Harris, J. (1985) *The Value of Life*. Routledge & Kegan Paul.

Illich, I. (1975) *Limits to Medicine*. Penguin.

Innes, H. Pearse and Crocker, L.H. (1985) (2nd Edition). *The Peckham Experiment*, Scottish Academic Press, Edinburgh.

Institute of Medical Ethics (1987) *Report of a Working Party on the Teaching of Medical Ethics* (The Pond Report). IME Publications.

Kant, I. (1974-7) *Works*. Suhkamp Taschenbucher.

Katch, F. I., and McArdle, W. D. (1983) *Nutrition, Weight Control and Exercise*. Lea & Febiger.

Kennedy, I. (1981) *The Unmasking of Medicine*. Allen & Unwin.

Kenny, A. J. P. (1978) *Freewill and Responsibility*. Routledge & Kegan Paul.

Kind, P., Rosser, R., and Williams, A. (1982) 'Valuation of quality of life: some psychometric evidence', in M. W. Jones-Lee (ed.) *The Value of Life and Safety*, North-Holland Publishing Co.

Kuhn, T. S. (1970) *The Structure of Scientific Revolutions*. University of Chicago Press.

Kuhn, T. S. (1977) *The Essential Tension: Selected Studies in Scientific Tradition and Change*. University of Chicago Press.

Lakatos, I., and Musgrove, A. (1970) *Criticism and the Growth of Knowledge*. Cambridge University Press.

Lawden, D. F. (1985) *Elements of Relativity Theory*. Wiley.

Lenthard, A. (1985) 'Well women centres: concepts and confusions', Polytechnic of the South Bank, London (unpublished).

Locke, J. (1984) *An Essay Concerning Human Understanding*. Oxford University Press.

Lockwood, M. (ed.) (1985) *Moral Dilemmas in Modern Medicine*. Oxford University Press.

Mill, J. S. (1910) *Utilitarianism, Liberty and Representative Government*. Dent.

Miller, D. (1976) *Social Justice*. Clarendon Press.

Moore, G. E. (1903) *Principia Ethica*. Cambridge University Press.

Office of Health Economics (1974) *Vaccination*. Office of Health Economics, London.

Pioneer Health Centre (1938) *Biologists in Search of Material: An Interim Report on the Work of the Pioneer Health Centre, Peckham*. Faber.

Plato (1986) *The Republic*, Penguin (Reprint).

Rachels, J. (1986) *The End of Life: Euthanasia and Morality*. Oxford University Press.

Raphael, D. D. (1981) *Moral Philosophy*. Oxford University Press.

Rawls, J. (1973) *A Theory of Justice*. Oxford University Press.

Seedhouse, D. (1984) 'Rationality'. PhD Thesis, Manchester University.

Seedhouse, D. (1986) *Health: The Foundations for Achievement*. Wiley.

Seedhouse, D., and Cribb, A. (eds.) (1988) *Changing Health Care*. Wiley (in press).

Stanley, I. M., Webster, C. A., and Webster, J. (1985) 'Comparative rating of consultation performance: a preliminary study and proposal for collaborative research', *Journal of the Royal College of General Practitioners*, **35**, 375–80.

Thompson, E. P. (1985) 'The transforming power of the cross', in R. Bocock and K. Thompson (eds.) *Religion and Ideology*. Manchester University Press.

United Kingdom Central Council for Nursing, Midwifery, and Health Visiting (1986) *Project 2000*.

Warnock, G. J. (1971) *The Object of Morality*. Methuen.

Warnock, M. (1978) *Ethics Since 1900*. Oxford University Press.

West, R., and Trevelyan, J. E. (1985) *Alternative Medicine: A Bibliography of Books in English*. Mansell.

WHO (World Health Organization) (1986) *Ottawa Charter for Health Promotion*. WHO.

Williams, A. (1985) 'Economics of coronary artery bypass grafting', *British Medical Journal*, **291**.

Wilson, M. (1976) 'Health enhancement or disease eradication', *Journal of the Institute of Health Education*, **14** (3), 75.

Wolf, F. A. (1981) *Taking the Quantum Leap*. Harper & Row.

Wyndham, J. (1959) 'Opposite number', in *The Seeds of Time*. Penguin.

Index